PASSIONATE
NUTRITION

A Guide to Using Food as Medicine from a Nutritionist
Who Healed Herself from the Inside Out

PASSIONATE
NUTRITION

A Guide to Using Food as Medicine from a Nutritionist
Who Healed Herself from the Inside Out

JENNIFER ADLER, MS, CN
with Jess Thomson

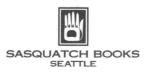

SASQUATCH BOOKS
SEATTLE

Printed in the United States of America

Published by Sasquatch Books

18 17 16 15 14   9 8 7 6 5 4 3 2 1

Editor: Susan Roxborough
Project editors: Michelle Hope Anderson & Nancy W. Cortelyou
Design: Joyce Hwang
Copy editor: Diane Sepanski
Writer: Jess Thomson
Cover photograph: Michelle Moore

Library of Congress Cataloging-in-Publication Data is available.

ISBN: 978-1-57061-945-8

Sasquatch Books
1904 Third Avenue, Suite 710
Seattle, WA 98101
(206) 467-4300
www.sasquatchbooks.com
custserv@sasquatchbooks.com

Page 119: Where Calories Go, Source: *Winning the War Within*,
Eileen Stellefson Myers, MPH, RDN, FADA,
copyright 2008: Used by permission of Helm Publishing Inc.

*Please note that the suggestions in this book are not meant to replace the proper
role of a reader's own nutritionists, doctors, or other health care providers. If you
think you may have a serious problem, please seek professional help.*

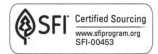

For my mother

CONTENTS

RECIPE LIST

ACKNOWLEDGMENTS

First, I'd like to express the deepest gratitude to Brené Brown, Ellyn Satter, Evelyn Tribole, Marc David, Sandor Ellix Katz, Sally Fallon, Geneen Roth, Weston Price, Susun Weed, Michael Gershon, Adelle Davis, Linda Bacon, and all the other leaders and researchers quoted in these pages. Your wisdom and studies have formed the foundation of my practice, and without them I couldn't have built Passionate Nutrition into what it is today. I'd also like to offer sincere thanks to the following:

To Byron Katie, for changing my life.

To Jon, my husband, for his encouragement and wisdom. His love and inspiration helped make this book what it is.

To Jess Thomson, my cowriter, for being an incredible wordsmith and partner. You define grace under pressure.

To researcher and nutritionist Emily Ziedman, my tireless assistant, thank you for helping with the legwork required for the book. You are my second set of eyes.

To the wise women of Passionate Nutrition, for their thoughtful work with clients, and willingness to build the dream together.

To Ritzy Ryciak, for the inspiration for this book.

To David Wiseman, for being there since the beginning.

To Kimberly, my loving sister, for all our shared memories.

To Irene King, for being my heart and anchor.

To Cynthia Lair, for believing in me and being a tireless advocate for the whole foods movement.

To Bill Gottleib, for advice and support.

To Sue Bates, for her introduction to the world of eating disorders.

To Jayne Halsey, for helping me learn to define "healthy."

To all my clients and friends who have trusted me over the years, for sharing with me the intimacy of what they eat.

Acknowledgments

To Amie McCampbell and Mark Cohen, for taking the time to send interesting research my way.

To the book's early readers, who offered insight, clarity, and assistance: Maggie Kemper Rogers, Lindsay Simpson, Hilary Halttunen, Rebekah Denn, Amy Howe, Heather Thomson, Tracy Erbeck, and Ross Kane.

To the countless farmers, purveyors, consumers, and advocates who are dedicating their lives to bringing whole foods back to the table.

To Maureen and Barry Christ, for sharing their house with us.

To Michelle Moore, who took the photo on the cover.

To the estimable team who helped make this book a reality: Gary Luke at Sasquatch Books; editors Susan Roxborough, Nancy Cortelyou, and Michelle Hope Anderson; marketing team Sarah Hanson and Haley Stocking; copy editor Diane Sepanski; and designer Joyce Hwang helped shape it into something one big step better than I ever imagined it being. Thank you for believing in me and being so constantly supportive.

To all the clients and friends who have trusted me over the years, for sharing with me the intimacy of what they eat, and to those who allowed me to use their testimonials in these pages: Anne Pomerantz, Laurie McCauley, Debi Carpenter, Adrienne Bloom, Rachael Alnwick, Stand, Cindy Lovell, Cheryl Marks, Janette Ahrndt, Joan Krussel, Donna Huss, Amy Gooden, Helen Tapping, M.R. Olhava, Cheryl Quinn, and Anna Sabey, plus handfuls of those who chose to remain anonymous.

And to my mother, for asking me to find a way to make the world a better place. This book is for you, and for the wise women who have led the way before me.

INTRODUCTION

Reality is always the story of the past,
and what I like about the past is—it's over.

—Byron Katie

Look at me. Go ahead—take a good, long look. (I won't mind—I'm stuck on the cover.) I'm forty, but I don't have noticeable wrinkles. The skin under my eyes is the same texture and color as the skin on my cheeks. My hair could qualify me for a shampoo commercial. I look more like the owner of a successful nutrition-consulting practice than the poster child of poverty and struggle, but I spent my first two decades hungry, malnourished, and neglected. By age twenty, I'd suffered the catalog of illnesses that plague the poor: malnutrition, heavy-metal toxicity, parasites, anemia, hypoglycemia, and debilitating digestive disorders. When my mother died of cancer in her early forties, I realized I had two options: I could suffer a short, painful life, as she had, or make a monumental change and overhaul my lifestyle. I began a journey back to health using food as medicine, learning through a graduate degree in nutrition, extensive world travel, and living off the grid that what we eat plays a powerful role in healing. This book shares my story and the wisdom I've learned along the way.

Today I am the woman on the cover, but I probably don't eat what you'd guess. I don't buy low-fat anything. I eat my salad with dressing, every time. I use a full stick of butter to roast a chicken (see page 230), and yes, I eat the skin—often before the chicken gets to the table. I believe that foods aren't inherently good or bad; rather, it's our relationship with them that determines their meaning. Eating is something we do multiple times a day, every day of our lives, so if we're stressed about what we're eating or not eating, we're stressed every single day, all day long.

For that reason—and for many, many others—it's important for me to emphasize that this is a book about your *diet*, but it's not about *dieting*. It's about adding the right foods to your day instead of taking foods away, and eating things made with ingredients your grandmother knew. It's about stopping the painful, ineffective dieting cycle so many of us have suffered and using self-respect, self-confidence, self-knowledge, and self-love, instead of media and advertising, to make our food choices.

There's a good chance you're like many of my clients, who have come to Passionate Nutrition since its founding in 2003 in search of a variety of answers, with one common theme: You want to lose weight, and you want sustainable success. You want to feel better, and you want it to last. Watching clients make positive changes to the way they eat and the way they feel about their bodies has been exceptionally rewarding. But as a nutritionist whose role often skews toward teacher, it's frustrated me that my reach is limited to the women and men who walk through my doors. This book is for those who can't. It's my nutrition practice on paper. It's the story I tell my clients when they come in search of hope and confidence, but this time, it's told through the lens of my personal history.

This book is also a resource. I'll teach you the most important tenets of my nutrition practice, which range from emphasizing the importance of beneficial gut bacteria in digestion to using history as a dietary guide and understanding what causes sugar cravings. You'll learn why "health food" is a ridiculous term—shouldn't most things we put into our bodies be healthy?—and how much you really know about nutrition already. (To start, take the Do You Know Nutrition? quiz on page 23.) In Part IV, you'll find recipes for the ingredients I rely on that you might not be as familiar with in your kitchen—things like kimchi, kefir, sardines, nettles, organ meats, seaweed, and real fats.

If someone like my desperate twenty-year-old self walked into my office today, I would tell her to open up her medicine cabinet and sweep her bottles of pills and supplements into a trash bag. I would explain that, while medication has its place, a change in diet is usually far more powerful. I would reassure her that despite how she felt—lost, hungry, frustrated, bloated, cramped, and tired—she wasn't alone. I'd emphasize that she's not seeing symptoms of an existential character defect, but of a flawed food and health culture that does not support healthy eating habits. I'd teach her that digestion is the foundation of health and show her how changing what happens before and after she swallows can transform her life. I'd hold her hand and tell her she could heal. And then I'd show her how.

In this book, I discuss the food we eat and why we eat it. I emphasize abundance and joyful eating over restriction. I talk about weight loss, but I mostly talk about feeling better and looking better. My goal is to help you create your own personal food philosophy—one that works for you, on your terms, in your life. Take what resonates with you and leave the rest.

I start with my own story, as both a means of explaining where I come from and, I hope, a way to show why I believe everyone is capable of change. The words may surprise you—I grew up partly in an abandoned gas station with a convicted criminal for a father and a depressed mother, and stole during my teen years to feed myself and my sister—but this is my true story. (None of my clients and few of my friends know this story.) You'll learn why nutrition became my passion. You'll see how I regenerated my body, my life, and my spirit. And ultimately, you'll be able to transform your own life, as different as it may be, in an enjoyable, sustainable way.

Part I

THE BACKGROUND

Chapter 1

MY STORY

*People from the most horrendous of childhoods
can have good lives, but it comes down to a very
seemingly simple word. "Choice."*

—Dr. Laura Schlessinger

I start this book with my story for two reasons. First, I tell it so you can see why I mean it when I say that from a nutritional perspective, I accept people as they are and meet them wherever they need to start. I started at zero—or maybe below zero, if that's possible. I am in no position to judge anyone by what they put in their mouth, so I don't. Second, I share it to illustrate how powerful food can be in healing the body.

I know you have a story too. Maybe it's weight gain or an eating disorder. Maybe it's cancer. Maybe it's high blood pressure, allergies, depression, or any number of assorted conditions ranging from annoying to life threatening. Maybe you have circled around and around with different diets, trying one after the other, gaining hope for brief periods but eventually settling into the inevitable onset of failure. I've been there, and now, having found a long-term, sustainable approach to health and wellness, I'm the woman on the cover. I want to show you the hope you need to strive for change, and I want to give you the confidence that can get you there.

Missouri

Growing up, my parents didn't often use my name. It was just "Kid" or "Hey, kid," barked the way a stranger yells at a child who's wandering too close to the edge of a pool. Perhaps, in their own intuitive way, my parents knew that how they were raising my sister and me was akin to that. In that case, it was a deep, murky, dangerous pool, and there was no lifeguard.

My earliest memory is from age four, when my father, evading criminal charges for burglary, moved my mother and me from military housing in New Mexico to an abandoned gas station in Missouri. My sister Kimberly was born soon after. I remember the way my dad's *Playboy* magazines towered in stacks in the windows, how we used to ride our trikes around in circles inside, and how Dad would cut up old tires to patch the bottoms of our shoes. I didn't have *Brady Bunch* worries, like who stayed on the telephone too long or how many vegetables we had to eat. I don't remember having vegetables.

I don't have many happy memories from my childhood, either. In addition to being a thief, my father was a convicted pedophile; he was also sexually and emotionally abusive to his family. The places I remember most fondly are the safe, quiet places I chose for crying—places like the school library, where I'd often hide, alone, between the bookshelves in the back, or the brush pile in the trees behind the gas station, where I befriended feral cats. Being alone in the dark woods, in the solitude of nature, was my safe haven. I remember my sister from those early years, but I don't remember playing with her. I don't think we played, in the normal kid sense. We survived, with Led Zeppelin blaring in the background.

4

We lived off Malt-O-Meal and whatever Dad shot and killed that day, when he wasn't working. We were a perfect picture of rural poverty.

Pennsylvania

When I was ten, we moved and lived for a brief time in Pennsylvania, where my father was incarcerated again—not for stealing this time or for harming my sister and me, but for abusing young boys. My mother took over as our primary caretaker, but she was disabled by something none of us could identify—a depression that left her withdrawn and quiet, a shell of a woman who'd been beaten down too long. My sister and I, alone most of the time, remember deep, daily hunger pains. Our monthly trips to the grocery store stopped. There was no such thing as dinnertime. We attended school, but we didn't get the free lunches available to families with financial struggles. We certainly qualified, but no one bothered to fill out the paperwork. Malnourished and weak, we often ended up in the school nurse's office, where one official or another would call my mother and request we be taken home to recover from whatever illness we'd acquired. Breakfast was nonexistent. I don't remember eating—in fact, I don't remember much about this time in my life, especially compared to my sister, who seems to remember every detail—but I do remember hiding in the small room where we had a television. I remember being very scared.

At the time, I was constantly sick. If I had a sleepover with school friends, I knew I'd be sick for days, because my body was always too depleted to handle new germs or fatigue. I couldn't do what other kids could do. My mother was attentive when she was around, but she worked constantly, so my sister and I developed a pattern of self-rule. I ate what I could, when I could—a slice of pizza at a friend's house here, a shared candy bar there. The neighbors sometimes brought us watery milk made from powder when Mom was working. I started noticing deep, stabbing pains in my back. We didn't see doctors at all, so there was no solution. Now I know they were kidney problems, likely caused by severe dehydration.

Los Angeles

The only thing we could depend on was change. After my father was released from jail in Pennsylvania, he moved to Los Angeles to find work. Emaciated, depressed, and inexplicably incapable, my mother put my five-year-old sister and me on an airplane to "visit" our father in California. When he refused to return us to Pennsylvania, my mother moved to Los Angeles as well, where she worked in a label factory.

One day she made a rare visit to the doctor, who diagnosed her with breast cancer. Dad drove Mom back to work immediately, to finish her shift, and then decided to run. My sister, elated, helped him pack his things into milk crates and shove them into his black Chevy Camaro. Not having our abusive father in the house relieved us of untold amounts of stress, but he left me, at age twelve, and my sister, age seven, to care for our mother, the household, and ourselves. The wheels came off the wagon.

Around this time, I started gravitating toward a bad crowd at school, but I also became my sister's main caretaker (and at times, my mother's). I learned to steal food to feed us. Candy bars and processed baked goods were our mainstays. Spoonfuls of mayonnaise, handfuls of raw oatmeal, and bites of raw ramen noodles were common dinner staples. We kept red buckets next to my mother's simple bed after her treatments. She'd spend days vomiting, and we'd return from school to empty the buckets and clean up after her as much as she would let us. (On one occasion, my sister accidentally dropped a dollar into the bucket, and had no choice but to dig it out for food.) Mom wasted away—first down to one hundred pounds, then down to eighty. We all avoided talking about it. Eventually—miraculously—the cancer went into remission.

Meanwhile, I became a teenager in an inner-city school with little supervision. Twelve is a young (but not uncommon) age to begin experimenting with alcohol and drugs, and experiment I did—with both, and theft, and sex. Seeing that my parenting skills were wanting, my mother had the good sense to send my sister to live with our father, who'd moved to a nearby suburb.

Since she realized I was too young to live without an adult in the house, she asked my eighteen-year-old alcoholic boyfriend to move in, so that she could in turn move in with her own boyfriend. That scenario went as expected, and eventually, I moved in with my father and sister.

I remember my junior high and high school years as the hungriest. We still didn't get free lunches at school, so I only ate when friends shared their lunch tickets with me. Once, I wound up in juvenile detention for stealing cars and robbing homes; I stayed for what felt like a week because no one could reach my family. But there, I had food. I remember that so clearly. They served ham-and-cheese sandwiches on white bread. Juvenile hall isn't a comfortable place, but having food delivered to me regularly made me almost feel like royalty. I remember a waterfall of calm washing over me as calories sated the frantic hunger sensations I'd become so accustomed to feeling.

My memories of that time are quite hazy. My father's method of controlling my drinking and drugging was to avoid the topic. My life wasn't safe. There were guns, razor blades, and tattoos involved. I always drank the inch of liquid at the bottom of other peoples' beers at parties. My body was once used in a satanic ritual, which I don't even remember clearly. At fifteen, like so many teenagers, I was angry with my mother for what I saw as her having abandoned us with the man she'd pledged to protect us from. I spiraled further downward. Considering my trajectory, a court-ordered rehabilitation program was imminent. I went to drug and alcohol treatment, but my father pulled me out of the program because, according to him, he didn't want to have to remove all the alcohol from the house, which was part of the deal. I fell immediately back into the same bad patterns and came close to overdosing on cocaine on countless occasions.

Still, part of me was living as a parent, responsible for the care and feeding of my sister, then eleven. I found my first job as a cashier at a 1950s-style, strip-mall hot dog and burger place, which allowed me to bring food home. (We ate a lot of french fries.) Because my life—incredibly—offered my sister more relative safety than she had at home with our father, whose actions were totally unpredictable, I took her everywhere I went. If I spent the night at a friend's house, she came. If I went to a punk-rock concert, she was there. She watched people get tattoos, shoot heroin, and run from gun violence on a regular basis before she hit puberty. I was furious with my mother.

Sweet sixteen was good to me. That spring, my father went to Malaysia to marry a woman he'd met at a garage sale, and I still wasn't on speaking terms with my mother, so I had the run of my father's apartment for a few weeks. And I was beginning to think about appliances, of all things. The stove/oven combo in our kitchen didn't work, but I decided, for reasons still unclear to me, that I wanted to be able to cook food for my sister. I'd worked enough to save the $200 I needed for a countertop oven. Strangely, I didn't really know what to do with it when we got it home. I don't even remember cooking anything beyond cake (from a box) in it, honestly. I think it was a symbol of finding a home, an attempt to ground us. We needed grounding.

There were still drugs, and lots of them. One day, my boyfriend, Brian, a Korean guy, asked me to stop taking them. He was a heavily tattooed gangster type—he'd hold a gun to my head and threaten to shoot me (or both of us) when he was mad or jealous—but he told me I was smart and had the potential to do something great with my life. His words rocked my world. At the time, my self-esteem was low enough that I clung to him, even after being shot at as we ducked behind car tires. He was the first person to give me positive, uplifting feedback about who I was. He helped me realize that my life could expand beyond drugs, alcohol, abuse, and crime.

Although I didn't quit using mood-altering substances immediately, he'd planted a seed. I graduated from a high school where watching *Nightline* qualified as history class. After graduation, I worked two night jobs—as a dancer and escort at Club Fantasy, a men's dance club in Los Angeles, and for UPS at the airport, loading large containers onto airplanes in the wee hours each morning—and enrolled in community college, hoping to transfer to a four-year university. Suddenly, I was crazy about school. Education seemed an obvious stepping-stone out of the ghetto. I took a full course load every semester and slept with earplugs in for a few hours each day.

By eighteen, my drug use had decreased dramatically, but I ran entirely on adrenaline, which was kind of a drug in itself. I don't really remember eating while I was in community college, beyond cake, french fries, and doughnuts. (I'm still a sucker for a good old-fashioned.) I was a shell of a person, running desperately between school and work and back again, doing what I thought was needed to escape the cycle of poverty and violence I'd grown accustomed to. It was during this period, living with Brian and selling my sex appeal to pay for school, that I started a lifetime habit of self-help. I'd listen religiously to psychologist and counselor Dr. Laura Schlessinger on the radio. I started reading her books. I learned that I wanted to heal. My mother apologized, and suddenly I had an ally again. We plotted to finish college together (she hadn't finished and we were interested in the same classes), and we both applied to the University of Nebraska at Kearney, near where my mother's family lived and where I had spent time as a small child.

Nebraska

Since I had finished two years of community college and my mother had previously completed two years of college, we enrolled at the same level, more or less—only my mother's cancer had returned, so my college experience was outlined by the shadow of illness. Everything in Nebraska, from the patterns in the dust to the color of the sky, seemed foreign. I would cry walking between classes because it was so cold. I watched my sister get pregnant at sixteen—she wanted to provide my mother with a grandchild before her death—because my mother had been given a limited time to live. Mom visited doctor after doctor, but as it became clear that she was going to die, I started hypothesizing that perhaps her lifetime of abuse and self-destruction—a pattern I had clearly imitated for many years—had ruined her body. I began connecting her body's desperation with her lack of nutritious food and decided that if modern medicine couldn't help her, food might. And I had the illusion that I was the one in charge.

I started with a trip to a health food store way outside our little nothing Nebraska town. It was a sad, dusty shop with half-stocked shelves that smelled like old tea and old women. I brought Mom awful-smelling dried seaweed and bottled supplements and teas—anything the clerk and I, combined with my extensive readings, thought might do her some good. A frantic search for information about nutrition and cancer consumed me. Mom tried anything I suggested.

As my mother's condition worsened, I decided to explore other options. I'd found a job with an airline that gave me travel benefits, and waited tables at night, saving as much as I could to get away. I bought a plane ticket to Ecuador and Peru, leaving when my mother was in a stable period with $400 in my pocket and the vague notion that the region's jungles were the birthplace of much of our natural medicine. I can't say I was looking for a breast cancer cure, but I was certainly open to finding information that seemed to evade me at the local library.

That first nutrition-focused trip was really more of a wander. I traveled absurdly inexpensively, sometimes sleeping in dreadful hostels and eating what the poorest locals ate. But I noticed that what I could afford—fruits and vegetables and hot foods, like potatoes, corn, and quinoa, from small market stands—was the same food the local elders seemed to be eating. The food was simple and cheap, but the people were strong. It was the first time I connected health with simple, natural food, the first time my diet didn't come largely out of a package.

Unfortunately, I also wasn't very careful about which market stands I chose. I spent a day under a tree near Machu Picchu because I was too sick to function and returned to the States with a host of parasites impermeable to antibiotics and any other form of treatment I could find.

Aspen

When I returned, filled with hope for my mother (whose health had been improving steadily) and a stomach full of trouble, I decided to move to

Aspen, Colorado, where a friend I'd met while traveling was living. I worked as a ski lift operator, which provided me with housing, and as a server at The Little Nell, a five-star restaurant at the base of Aspen Mountain, which provided me with the notion that I was starting to know something about food. I kept tabs on my mother, who seemed to be defying all odds, my sister, and my newborn nephew from afar, and turned toward an extremely simple life.

My foods were still limited—not because I was trying to curb my intake or focus on certain nutrients, but because back in the United States, I didn't have a food vocabulary beyond french fries, sweets, and the occasional slice of pizza. Among friends, I was known as the gassy girl, the one always dealing with digestive stress. I laughed it off in public, but in private, there was a lot of pain involved. Every time I ate, I became bloated and cramped. I did my best to ignore my body.

When the snow season ended, I took a job as a nanny for an extraordinarily wealthy family who initially had no idea I had no cooking, cleaning, or child-care skills. (Somewhere along the way, I'd learned that I could convince people I had experience in almost anything. My time in Aspen was the pinnacle of that.) I had a lovely room in the basement of their slopeside mansion. In very little time, my employer figured out that I was clueless but hard working; she taught me how to make beds and clean properly, and that putting dinner on the table meant an array of things—protein *and* vegetables, for example. She introduced me to the concept of dinner as a place where people sit down to eat together.

My mother's health declined, again. This time, she decided to move near me. She rented a space in Basalt, Colorado, a town about twenty minutes away, where she wilted. I saw her only occasionally because I was working two full-time jobs. Truthfully, I didn't realize how sick she was. One day, I returned from a backpacking trip to discover she'd been transferred to the intensive care unit at the Aspen hospital. She was clearly nearing the end of her life and needed to be back in Nebraska, where extended family could care for her on a regular, long-term basis. She was also clearly too weak to travel. My employer—a woman whose kindness I'll never forget—flew Mom back to Nebraska on her private jet. A few months later, after many iterations of moving back and forth between Nebraska and Aspen to help care for my mom, I followed.

Nebraska, Again

At my grandparents' house, I sat with my mother through the pain as her cancer metastasized. She moved to a hospital, where she suffered her first grand mal seizure—obviously horrific for her, but it was also traumatic for me—and asked me to change the food hospitals serve their patients. The next months were painful on all levels. Knowing she didn't have much time left, my mother apologized for, in her words, being a "bad" mother. I forgave her because I knew she had done the best she could.

Her seizures intensified, and the cancer spread to her bones, making them brittle enough to break regularly. (She was allergic to morphine, and the doctors were never able to get her pain under control. My sister, who not coincidentally now works in hospice as a Certified Nursing Assistant, says people no longer die like our mother died.) As her body disintegrated, I started contemplating a graduate school program in nutrition. By the spring of 2000, she was gone. In the end, I knew that even with the limited nutritional information I had, I'd improved her quality of life until her last breath. On her deathbed, I vowed to go back to school.

I applied and was accepted to Seattle's Bastyr University with an admissions essay that detailed my journey with my mom. I spent a month traveling in Morocco, cruising the spice shops and bazaars. There, it baffled me that an entire culture seemed to solve their ills with spices—cumin to cure morning sickness, cinnamon to aid digestion, nigella seeds for joint pain, turmeric to stop bleeding. Although I hadn't yet realized that I loved traveling in part because I ate foods abroad that were good for my body, I started latching on to the concept that I could control how my stomach felt by eating differently. I moved back to the States prepared to learn as much as I could about nutrition.

Seattle

After a summer studying chemistry to catch up with the other matriculating students, I landed in Seattle. Ironically, my years at Bastyr, where I received a master's degree in Clinical Nutritional Counseling, coincided with my most physically painful years. By 2000, I'd recognized that eating certain foods exacerbated the digestive issues I'd been having (which I'll discuss in more detail in Chapter 4). Based on the food-eliminating diets I'd learned about at Bastyr, I was living on pears, oatmeal, and cashews, with a few other occasional foods. I slept twelve to fourteen hours every night, exhausted by pain and discomfort, and spent my waking time at school. I gleaned information from peers at the local food co-op, where I taught nutrition classes, and at the university's medicinal herb garden, where I also worked.

It wasn't until I was actually immersed in a nutrition program that I began to fully understand I needed to eat fruits and vegetables, but in my mind then, they had to be raw. After a decade of vegetarianism—my father's hunting habits and my love for animals had turned me off meat as a young teen—I realized I needed more protein. I read book after book, but it seemed like everything I was reading was a contradiction: *Eat mostly meat. Eat only vegetables. Eat three meals a day. Eat only small meals throughout the day.* I became more and more confused, and my digestion was actually getting worse.

Looking for a more effective approach to calming my digestive tract, I began to intensively research ethnic approaches to healing. I traveled to Japan, where I learned how miso can be soothing and how the minerals in seaweed can nourish the body. Studying Ayurvedic medicine in India was also eye opening, but not because I started eating according to the *dosha*, or body type, the practice prescribes. Rather, in India, I was terrified of eating something that would make me sick, so I ate only foods that were super-cooked. For the first time in my adult life, I became capable of eating without pain.

Coming home after my travels, my body began to calm down. I started experimenting with cooking more, adding new foods to my diet that didn't necessarily match what I'd learned in my nutrition courses. Ultimately I learned that my health depended on listening to my own body's needs, rather than the needs prescribed by fad diets or nutrition textbooks. I discovered that being a good nutritionist sometimes requires forgetting all about nutrition. Sometimes, a body just needs to eat.

Ward, Colorado

Although I didn't agree wholeheartedly with everything I'd learned at Bastyr, it remained clear to me that I could teach people about using food as medicine. The problem was, I still didn't really know how to cook. I ate functionally, choosing the foods that made my body feel good, but I wanted to know how to make food taste good. I enrolled in a natural-foods cooking school in Boulder, Colorado. Still financially tied to my sister (and perpetually terrified of homelessness), I found the cheapest lodging I could: I lived for free in an eight-by-eight-foot cabin owned by a friend of a friend in Ward, a tiny, self-governed hippie town forty-five minutes from Boulder.

In Ward, I went through multiple personal revolutions. First, in the cabin I became completely independent, living off the grid and alone. The woods became my safe haven, as they had been in my childhood. Late nights after school, I journaled and read, and really sat still to think for the first time. I began to work through my mother's death, which helped lift me out of the depression that had consumed me in Seattle, and I recognized that the goofy, fluttery feelings I had around a female friend in Boulder might be sexual. I came out as a lesbian and began to feel a sense of freedom from the sexual abuse I had endured as a child and teenager—by my father, and by other men, while I was under the influence of drugs and alcohol.

Culinary school changed two major things about the way I was eating: vegetables started tasting good, and meat became part of my diet again. Every morning, after an early lecture, we'd gather in a small, cramped kitchen, where a flighty teacher with a lot of burn scars coached us on cooking intuitively. She taught us to use recipes only as guides and instead emphasized cooking through our senses of smell and taste. I ate well at school every day. My gassiness decreased every week. Mentally, I became less afraid of eating—less afraid of what it might do to me.

Whether my sudden happiness and health in Colorado depended on sexual emancipation or simply eating well isn't clear, but I knew then—as I know now—that both were important. Both decreased my stress enormously. I finished school with a renewed drive to start a nutrition practice. I wanted to teach people to find their own path out of pain the way I had.

Seattle, Again

When cooking school ended, Seattle called. I sold my bike to rent an attic to live in. At first, I worked as a colon hydrotherapist to pay the bills. My first real love, Suzanna, and I moved in together, eventually living off the grid on Vashon Island, a quick ferry ride from Seattle. Soon, I founded a nutrition practice in Seattle's Pioneer Square neighborhood. I called it Realize Health because it seemed like so many people walked around simply not realizing that they could feel better if they ate differently. At first, my practice was tiny. I slept in my office to save the ferry fare when it made sense, and spent every possible hour teaching classes and giving nutrition talks to promote the business. We lived very inexpensively and prioritized travel, education, and food. As money began to come in, I looked for more knowledge; I studied how food played a part in healing in China, Belize, Guatemala, and Mexico.

Around 2008, things started changing very quickly for me. Suzanna and I separated, and my sister needed to get out of an abusive relationship with an alcoholic man, so I again began supporting her. Kimberly moved to Seattle with her three children, and we've mostly lived together since then. Needless to say, supporting five people with my sole income became slightly more challenging than supporting just myself.

I also resolved to make peace with my past and signed up for the nine-day School for The Work with Byron Katie, a world-renowned writer and teacher who shows people how to identify and question the thoughts that cause all suffering. It wouldn't be an exaggeration to call my time with her life-changing. Perhaps most importantly, she helped me assess my issues with men. Years of working as an escort had left me with a constant, inescapable shame about myself and my body, and a fear of people learning that I'd been paid for sex. I felt that because I had made those choices as a consensual adult, I was tainted and unworthy.

The nine days also helped calm the more irrational fears I'd developed over the course of my life: fears of being homeless and going hungry, of dying of cancer, of being unable to take care of my sister and her children. Doing The Work helped me accept my past in a rational way and taught me how, instead of ignoring it or trying to escape it, I could use it to form and inform my future. I learned to question my negative thoughts; I started looking at my past as a blessing and now see it as an inspiration.

My business also changed dramatically. As I learned more about my own approach to eating and realized that I was more excited about nutrition than most typical clinicians, I changed my practice's name to Passionate Nutrition. Clients poured in, and I started bringing on additional staff. I became known as the nutritionist who could also seamlessly incorporate the often-psychological aspects of eating. People came in because I was reputed to be nonjudgmental. While I never claim or intend to be a mental or emotional health expert, it's clear that my own path to healing—physically, from the effects of malnutrition, and emotionally, from abuse—has given me the groundwork necessary to teach others to do the same.

In 2010, I met Jon. That summer, as a direct result of my work with Byron Katie, we married, blending his family with mine, which still included my sister and her children. He shows me love and unending acceptance. I could not possibly have found a better match.

Today, Passionate Nutrition has grown to include more than twenty offices, thirty-six practitioners, and four personal chefs. We've seen thousands of clients over the course of more than twenty thousand visits. I feel I owe my success to extremes. I went from Snickers to seaweed, from foraging for a dollar bill in a bucket to foraging for power foods in the forest along the Pacific coast. My path cut from experiencing nutritional deprivation to thriving on nutrient-dense meals; from harboring global human distrust to hosting a web of loving, trusting relationships; from suffering from poor health to waking with a vibrant energy and sense of well-being totally foreign to me as a child and young adult.

Today, when someone calls me "Jennifer" instead of "Hey, kid," like my parents did, I still do a little bit of a double take, because it seems like such a personal way to approach a person. In public, and in this book, I still call Kimberly "my sister," because that's what I grew up with. She didn't have a first name, either. If someone had told me, at age fourteen or so, that I'd grow up to help people heal their bodies with food, I'd probably have cried.

Today, I'm still a crier. I cry for different reasons, though: for the homeless guy on the street, for the kid in the soap commercial, and for the photos of cats at the adoption center. I'm sensitive. But I no longer cry because I'm hungry or because eating causes me emotional or physical pain. Neither should you.

Chapter 2

YOUR STORY

*We are all wonderful, beautiful wrecks. That's
what connects us—that we're all broken, all
beautifully imperfect.*

—Emilio Estevez

When a client calls me for the first time, they often don't know what questions to ask. They stammer, because they're nervous to admit they're unhappy with their weight or that they need guidance, and because they honestly doubt there is new and exciting information a nutritionist can give them. They've tried everything possible to look and feel better. They've read magazine articles and best-selling books about the latest diets. They've gone through spouses, houses, and jobs, but the excess weight or physical malady that's plagued them for decades won't go away. Nothing has worked, and they have often begun isolating themselves due to depression, shame, and unavoidable temptation. They are utterly broken.

Chances are you won't have the same history I do, but perhaps we've felt similarly. In 2000, I didn't have the energy for life; I was eating just pears, cashews, and oatmeal in an attempt to calm my riotous digestive system. Eating caused me debilitating physical pain, but there was emotional pain too. I began to hate food. I grieved for the health I might have had, had I grown up differently. I felt guilty that I couldn't make myself better. I recovered by changing my relationship with food, and learning to use it to heal. Over the last decade, I've taught others to do the same.

The core of what I do revolves not just around food, but around our relationship with it. Based on years of research, my own experience and that of my clients, and common sense, I've developed an approach to healthy living that relies heavily on Byron Katie's book *Loving What Is*, which leads to self-acceptance and "loving what is," listening to our innate body wisdom, and moving away from the fears we have surrounding food. For many people, a glimpse of the refrigerator causes a whirlwind of negative emotions such as fear, guilt, heartbreak, sadness, panic, and disappointment. I want to replace those feelings—and the inevitable sense of failure that so many of those who have tried to lose weight can't avoid—with a habit of eating abundantly and approaching food positively.

If you walk through my door looking for weight loss, like 80 percent of my clients do, the hardest thing I'll ask you to do the first day is list what you've done to promote your own health that week. Most people, having been conditioned to accept that being overweight or in some way unhealthy means they have some inherent character flaw, aren't ready to talk about what they're doing right. They think about the failures—years and years of trying to look and feel better without success. You've probably experienced the same desperation, the same constant exasperation. But if you're reading this, you're already on the right path.

I'll also ask you if you know when you're hungry and what foods you crave. I'll ask not just what you eat, but who you eat it with and how—and your answers will tell me much more about what you need than just learning what you ate that week ever could. We'll start by balancing your physiology, building a good foundation of health in your gut, and making sure you're getting the nutrients you need. Slowly, once your body feels more balanced, we will address the emotional aspects of eating.

What Are You Doing Right?

Most of us spend plenty of energy regurgitating negative thoughts, but forget to recognize and honor the positive things we do for ourselves. Start putting this book into action by listing three positive things you do for yourself every week. Examples might include drinking water at work, eating breakfast more days than not, cooking a nice dinner for yourself at home on Friday, going for a walk with a neighbor, or stopping to eat lunch without distractions on a busy day. It could even be eating a so-called forbidden food with consciousness and enjoyment, and without beating yourself up.

Of course we'll talk about food, but the average person who sees me is confused about what the word "nutrition" means. (Do you know nutrition? Take the quiz on page 23. The answers might surprise you, especially if you, like so many of our clients, have been watching what you eat for years.) It's no wonder; popular fad diets replace previous ones faster than we can read about them. The word "nutrition" morphs every time we read the newspaper. Best-selling books contradict each other over major nutritional points, and randomized, double-blind, peer-reviewed, evidence-based research studies are validated, then proven wrong, every week. Anyone who's thought about trying to lose weight or eat differently with the goal of improving health has ridden a dietary roller coaster. It weaves through the sections at the grocery store, touting one aisle or another as "nutritious" or not, zooming through the fat-free yogurt section and pausing at the grapefruit bins, only to go around again as the trends recirculate. At Passionate Nutrition, we think the roller coaster just makes you sick.

This chapter explains the sane, natural, intuitive approach I take to health and healing at Passionate Nutrition. I don't want to offer a temporary patch, but rather, a permanent solution. This is the last nutrition book you'll need.

What I Believe

Clients come to Passionate Nutrition for a variety of reasons, but with one common goal: to feel better and continue feeling better. I believe we are successful partly because of the psychological approach to wellness mentioned before (and discussed in more detail in the pages that follow), but mostly because we teach clients to use food as medicine.

In the American medical community, it isn't common to rely on food to help people heal. Most gastroenterologists—doctors who study the digestive systems of people with problems such as irritable bowel syndrome and Crohn's disease—still don't connect their patients' disorders with what they put in their mouths. Rheumatologists don't advocate that arthritis patients eat anti-inflammatory foods to calm their joint pain. Students in medical school are typically offered just one nutrition course—and then only as an elective. In other words, there is no real connection in our medical communities between food and healing.

In my practice, I often aim to heal the same ailments but with a different approach—one that avoids supplements entirely, and instead relies solely on food.

Throughout history, food has been known to both prevent and cure many diseases, but because the food available to many American communities is usually poor, the system is inherently flawed. (Even well-intended institutional dietitians and nutritionists typically only have access to processed foods that are designed for long shelf lives and do little more than satisfy hunger, if that.) People are trying to heal with food that's been so altered it no longer qualifies as food. As a result, sick people are receiving an incomplete, sometimes incorrect, education about how eating can help

QUIZ: Do You Know Nutrition?

1. Losing weight is as simple as "calories in and calories out."

    a) True

    b) False

2. To be healthy and look young, we need to eat fat-free foods.

    a) True

    b) False

3. Raw food is always more nutritious than cooked food.

    a) True

    b) False

4. Which food provides the most potassium per serving?

    a) Banana

    b) Potato

    c) Dried apricot

    d) Salmon

5. Which of these foods can most effectively boost your metabolism?

    a) Acai berry

    b) Celery

    c) Seaweed

    d) Cayenne

6. Salt is bad for your health.

    a) True

    b) False

7. If you are focusing your budget on organic products that give you the biggest bang for your buck, which of the following would be most important?

   a) Vegetables
   b) Fruit
   c) Red meat
   d) Dairy
   e) C and D

8. Saturated fat is dangerous for your health.

   a) True
   b) False

9. Research has shown which of the following to be most addictive?

   a) Cocaine
   b) Morphine
   c) Sugar

10. Which of the following statements are true regarding grass-fed beef?

    a) Grass-fed beef has the same amount of fat as an equal portion of boneless, skinless chicken breast.
    b) Meat from grass-fed animals has two to four times more omega-3 fatty acids than meat from grain-fed animals.
    c) Grass-fed beef has lower levels of dietary cholesterol.
    d) Grass-fed beef has about twice the levels of conjugated linoleic acid, which may have cancer-fighting properties and lower the risk of diabetes and other health problems, than factory-raised beef.
    e) All of the above

11. Which of these foods has the most vitamin C?

    a) Oranges
    b) Cabbage
    c) Strawberries
    d) Bell peppers

12. Which of the following food has the most fiber?

    a) One avocado
    b) One slice whole-wheat bread
    c) One side garden salad
    d) One large peach

Please see page 243 for answers to the quiz.

them live longer, healthier lives. My typical day involves teaching people how to identify and eat "real" food—usually, the same kinds of things our grandmothers ate.

The practice of using food as medicine is sometimes referred to as "green medicine," but I just like to call it "eating." And I'm not the first. Stop and think about this: The body can't survive without food. Medicine is defined in *The Oxford English Dictionary* as "the science or practice of the diagnosis, treatment, and prevention of disease." So in a list of treatments and preventions, shouldn't what we can't survive without, what our body is made of, come first? If something's wrong with our skin, shouldn't we consider what forms that skin? Even Hippocrates, the ancient Greek physician, said, "Let food be thy medicine, and medicine be thy food." He died in 370 BC (at age ninety).

Of course, the degree to which people use and think of food as medicine varies. But studying nutrition around the globe regularly for two decades has taught me that Americans use food to treat various ailments far less than other cultures. In Japan, I visited Hiroshima, site of the 1945 atomic bombing, where I learned that instead of taking iodine tablets to ward off the effects of radiation sickness, as people did near Chernobyl, Japanese officials encouraged patients to ingest more seaweed because of its naturally high iodine levels. The seaweed also helped ward off autoimmune thyroid disease—a huge problem for people exposed to large amounts of radiation. They prescribed miso soup for the same issues.

In India, where foods are often very well cooked and/or fermented, I experienced firsthand how a change in eating practices can heal digestion. In both places, I noticed a common theme: There was no firm line between food and medicine. People ate what they needed, and from a healing perspective, digestion was considered paramount. Note that when you go to a Western medical clinic today, the doctor will immediately take your pulse and measure your blood pressure, then perhaps take blood to perform laboratory tests. But when was the last time your general practitioner asked you what your poop looks like? Ayurvedic and Chinese medicine practitioners rarely do labs; instead, they ask about digestion, including detailed information about a patient's stools. At Passionate Nutrition, we take the ancient approach, and after seeing thousands of clients experience dramatic, life-changing, long-term improvements, I think it's the best one.

Just as nutritious foods can make us well, unhealthy food (or lack of certain foods) can make us sick. Most chronic illnesses are born from nutritional deficiencies. It goes beyond scurvy, the disease caused by vitamin C deficiency famously suffered by sailors and explorers who didn't have access to fresh fruits and vegetables. Rosacea is often caused by a lack of hydrochloric acid, which the stomach produces in good health. Diabetes is most commonly caused by poor diet. Night blindness is primarily caused by a lack of vitamin A. Although there are clearly examples of sicknesses that require modern medication or various surgeries, much healing generally requires little more than nutritional support.

Ironically, in the United States, which the World Health Organization reported in 2012 spent more money per capita on health care than any other country, we eat the poorest-quality foods—foods that are overly processed, high in additives and preservatives, or tainted with pesticides, antibiotics, or hormones—and we suffer the effects. The US Department of Agriculture (USDA) reports that nutrient levels in the average fruits and vegetables have decreased upward of 30 percent in the last half century. The Centers for Disease Control and Prevention (CDC) also reports that the number of Americans with diabetes quadrupled between 1980 and 2012. The midcentury advent of Big Pharma and consequent marketing efforts aimed at designating pills as the answer to everything taught Americans over the course of the twentieth century that health comes from quick fixes, ready-made therapies, and fast foods. Recent generations have lost touch with the thousands of years' worth of food-as-medicine knowledge that our ancestors had. As a result, we are sicker than ever.

However, we may finally be "officially" learning that good nutrition— real food—can and should heal as effectively, if not *more* effectively, than some medicines. In 2007, the *Journal of Clinical Oncology* reported a higher breast cancer survival rate in active women with higher fruit and vegetable intake. In 2005, *The American Journal of Clinical Nutrition* said that oatmeal can be as effective in lowering cholesterol as initial doses of statin drugs (and without the nasty side effects). So-called power foods have started appearing in mainstream research too. For example, last year the *International Journal of Rheumatic Diseases* reported that sesame seeds can be more effective than Tylenol at relieving osteoarthritic knee pain. According to another 2013 study in the journal *Nutrition and Cancer*, edible red seaweed was more effective than tamoxifen, the leading mainstream drug, at suppressing cancerous tumor growth—without toxicity to the liver and kidneys. I believe in breaking the cultural habit of turning to medications first to heal our ills. In an almost spiritual way, I believe in eating.

Applying My Beliefs (Or, What I Do Differently)

Because I grew up in an unconventional way, it never occurred to me to be conventional in my approach to nutritional counseling. I will not make (or let) you count calories. I will ask you what foods you *like*. I'll give you a list of new foods to try. My methods stem from ancient forms of healing, which are quite typical in ethnic approaches to medicine, but my tactics might surprise you.

I'm not interested in telling people no when it comes to food. In my mind, limiting calories or fat, or telling people to forget about their favorite dessert, is restrictive fearmongering. Because it causes up-and-down craving cycles (which I cover in detail in Chapters 5 and 6), it's ineffective. It's also boring, and I believe that if what we eat three times a day or more is boring, our life suffers. Our life becomes boring. I teach people to avoid the black-and-white approach to choosing foods, and help erase the labels clients have about whether a food is intrinsically "good" or "bad."

Rather than deleting foods from your diet, I often start with adding foods you may be missing. Instead of preaching about eating more fruits and vegetables, I start by showing you strategies for correcting two physiological imbalances most of my clients suffer from: inadequate intestinal flora and inadequate protein. I talk about improving intestinal bacteria, which is the gut's most important arsenal for fighting disease and regulating digestion, in Chapter 4. Increasing protein intake, the subject of Chapter 5, often increases energy and decreases sugar cravings for clients almost immediately. For most people, adding the foods covered in these two chapters sets up a solid foundation for health.

As your body becomes more balanced, you naturally gravitate toward foods that sustain and heal you. The next part of my job, which I'll detail in Chapter 8, is helping you learn to listen to your body's natural wisdom. Note that the foods that work for you aren't necessarily the foods that work for your best friend, or your mother, or your children. Use a restaurant visit as an example: For most of us, when we sit down in front of a menu, there are usually one or two things that pop out as attractive right away. They are rarely the same things for everyone at the table because we all have our own intuition about what our bodies need. Teaching people that optimum health and wellness starts with listening to their own intelligent bodies— by doing things as simple as ordering that first thing that screams to them off the menu—is a crucial part of my practice. (About 80 percent of my clients come in for weight loss, so I know many are terrified by the prospect of letting their body take control. Trust me, you'll get there. By the time we get to Chapter 8, it will make sense.)

Typically, regardless of my client's initial goals, the results of applying these three simple but seemingly radical approaches—the eradication of the concept of "bad" foods, an increase in protein and beneficial bacteria consumption, and the acceptance of the body's own intelligence—are weight loss (intentional or not), increased energy, and a revitalized life. To my mind, this is the point at which I can help clients assess the issues they brought through the door. This is where sustainable change begins.

Regardless of why clients come into Passionate Nutrition, I share with them this list of beliefs that I consider the heart of my practice.

The Heart of Passionate Nutrition

A healthy diet relies on eating food that tastes good.
Deprivation does not work. As we become healthier, our bodies naturally gravitate away from "unhealthy" foods because the foods that taste good are the foods we need.

A healthy lifestyle is flexible and enjoyable.
I won't ask you to follow strict diets full of dos and don'ts and intense workout schedules. Instead, I will teach you the difference between cravings and true hunger, and introduce you to foods that will satisfy that hunger and help eliminate cravings.

When it comes to food, our ancestors knew what they were doing.
Ancient cultures developed successful food practices over thousands of years, understanding the value of certain foods, some of which have today become taboo, such as fatty and salty foods.

Shifting our focus to see what we are actively doing to support our health empowers us to make sustainable choices.
In America, we are shamed for eating cake or potato chips, or for flabby arms, love handles, acne, and even lack of energy. Many cultures don't have a translation for the word "should"—yet that one word rules how we live and what we eat. I'll help you discover what you're doing right so you can sidestep guilt and shame around eating.

The earth supplies us with an abundance of healthy foods designed to nourish body and soul.
When we listen to our body's messages, using my tools for tapping into body wisdom (see Chapter 8), and eat foods in their natural state, we tend to eat the portions we require and the foods we need.

Food is a gift meant to be savored and enjoyed.
Food is not meant to torment us. It's important to learn to approach food as a friend, not an enemy. Changes in our eating habits can lead to positive lifelong changes in how we feel and act.

Food is healing.
Rather than relying first on medicine to change the way we feel, Passionate Nutrition thinks food is the best medicine.

We all have the power to heal and transform our bodies.

Challenging Entrenched Beliefs

Whether consciously or not, each of us approaches food and diet according to a deeply engrained belief system that comes from a lifetime of eating—from how we ate as a child to what the latest trends and media messages condition us to believe. We carry this approach around, often more obviously on our sleeve than we realize.

It may seem strange, but after a decade of practicing, I can easily see what negative experiences and emotions most people carry around with them from the moment they walk into my office. People who are overly conscious of fat content and count calories obsessively will be quick-tempered, which makes sense; their nervous system isn't getting enough fat, so they are easily thrown into a state of anger. People who slump onto my couch with lifeless eyes and pale skin are often missing vitality because they eat a very functional, rigid, limited diet. They need spontaneity—spices, happy music while they're eating, new foods. In contrast, the person who walks in, grabs a croissant off the table, and digs in is a person who listens to her body and is able to accept the good things in life. She's probably pretty easy-going, relaxed, and fun to be around. A party of nutritionists, on the other hand, is likely to be as much fun as a root canal, because most of us have rigid, controlled rules about what's right and wrong regarding diet—rules that spill over into our lives, for better or worse. Over the years, I've been fairly accurate when I try to predict what challenges people might face. Throughout this book, I hope to change what you may think about nutritionists.

Regardless of who you are and what you'd do in my office, you likely need two things right now: hope and confidence. First, know that genetics play a role in what you look like and how your body acts, but they can be changed. According to Dr. José Ordovás, director of the Nutrition and Genomics Laboratory at Tufts University, genes contribute on average no more than 25 percent toward our total health picture. Ordovás argues that genetic makeup plays a relatively minor role in determining our destiny, especially compared to lifestyle factors like diet and exercise.

Know also that cells regenerate so fast that, as reported by Swedish stem cell biologist Dr. Jonas Frisén, the average age of all the cells in an adult human's body may be as young as seven years old—in any case, far younger than our chronological age. The cells that line the stomach regenerate every five days. Skin cells replace themselves almost as quickly. I embrace the possibility of change, which is why you—the one reading this book, hoping for change—can take control and direct your life's path in a monumental way. You are not a victim of your own body.

Bringing This Book Home

This book is different from my practice in one really significant way: I can't see you or talk to you. I can't watch your face when you talk about cake. I can't try to predict your emotional gustatory kryptonite. And perhaps most importantly, I can't close the door and encourage you to cry. At Passionate Nutrition, we go through two jumbo-size boxes of tissues every week in each of more than twenty offices. Clients often spend much of the first appointment or two in tears. When they feel sick, disappointed, or ashamed (or all three), it's hugely emotional for all of us. Initially, our job is to create a place of acceptance, understanding, and love, which is something we take great pride in—and something more difficult to do in the pages of a book.

Know that we understand you may feel terrified and frustrated. You may be, as they say, sick and tired of feeling sick and tired. You may be desperate, having tried and failed a variety of weight-loss or health strategies for decades. Chances are also good that you're very smart and well educated in the nutritional realm, having spent thousands of hours on the computer combing the web for nutrition information or advice on weight loss. (If research were the only criteria for a graduate degree in nutrition, you'd have probably earned a master's by now.) You may be angry about picking up a nutrition book in the first place, or perhaps thankful that ordering a book online meant you didn't have to leave your house.

However, regardless of who you are, what defines your personality, what genetics you were born with, or what food culture you were raised with, you have one thing in common with me and all of my other clients: We can all use food as medicine. Each of us can heal with food. We don't need a degree in food science or a book of ancient remedies. We do, however, need to be willing to make a few agreements with ourselves. We need to be ready for new patterns and new foods. Consider it an oath of sorts—let's call it The Oath of Openness (below). It's your decision whether to take it. Or maybe you'll just take some of it. It's your call.

The Oath of Openness

- I agree to let go of rigid beliefs about what is healthy or unhealthy when it comes to food.
- I will remain open to experimenting with the foods in this book, even if they are outside of my norm.
- I will give my body the time it needs to heal and repair. I know that my body is constantly regenerating itself, so healing is absolutely possible, but it takes time.
- I will listen to my body wisdom as I go through this transformation. My body knows what it needs and will steer me in the right direction.

I can tell you that if you follow the suggestions in this book that resonate with you, the results will rock your world. You'll attain your natural weight, your skin will glow, your hair will be full and shiny, the bags under your eyes will improve, the whites of your eyes will be whiter, your energy will increase, your bowel movements will become more regular, bloating after eating will cease, and aches and pains will lessen or disappear. There will be benefits on the cellular level also, including decreased inflammation and a stronger immune system. I list these things with such certainty because I've seen it work with thousands of clients. Of course, there are outliers—no nutritionist can claim to help 100 percent of her patients, typically because of extenuating health circumstances—but I like to think I come very close.

Eventually, you might also be angry. Many of my clients, after following the "rules" for years, some quite religiously, thinking they'd been eating well by limiting meats and fats and eating only raw vegetables, become profoundly upset when they begin to heal. They grieve the time, effort, and energy they wasted depriving themselves of the foods they love while still suffering health consequences. If food has been your friend and confidante, and it suddenly disappears or loses its charge as the thing you constantly obsess over, you'll need to find something new to do with the time and sanity you regain.

The Passionate Nutrition Timeline

The biggest misconception about healing is that it's instant. No instant change is sustainable. Below are the general steps I take to incorporate change into my clients' lives, and their associated timelines. As you can see, these timelines are fluid. What's right for you depends on who you are.

- Incorporating gut-strengthening foods: 1 to 12 weeks
- Balancing protein, fat, and caloric intake: 3 to 12 months
- Working on the emotional aspects of eating: 3 months to 2 years

Welcome to Passionate Nutrition

I'm not sure why you're reading this. We see all types of clients. Maybe you're struggling with those last ten pounds—real or imagined excess weight. You might be struggling with digestive issues, depression, anxiety, fatigue, cancer, diabetes, high blood pressure, high cholesterol, allergies, infertility, an eating disorder, or the effects of menopause. You might be confused by all the contradictory information about health, nutrition, and diet. You may have been on and off multiple diets and are fed up with feeling frustrated, discouraged, and furious because you can't seem to stay on the track you think is right. You may be a shameful eater who binges on low-fat or sugar-free foods and have lost all of the joy you once found in food. Maybe you simply want to feel better, or are too busy to eat healthy meals, or just want to feed your family well. In any case, you're not alone. Passionate Nutrition sees hundreds like you every week. I was once in a similar place.

But now you're here, which means that you'll learn a host of tried-and-true methods for regaining and maintaining your health once and for all. I'll show you why and how our food culture is flawed. I'll help you stabilize your relationship with food. And you'll heal using food—"forbidden" foods, nutrient-dense foods, new foods, and old foods, made with recipes that span the ages—so that it becomes a source of healing rather than pain.

Welcome to Passionate Nutrition.

Part II

THE BASICS

Chapter 3

THE 100-YEAR DIET

*The food you eat can be either the safest and most
powerful form of medicine or the slowest form of poison.*

—Dr. Ann Wigmore, ND

I'm a bit of a burger connoisseur. At Bainbridge Island's Harbour Public House, my go-to spot close to home, the burgers come big and sloppy. I like the Seoul Burger, which is piled with house-made kimchi. And as a nutritionist, I believe it's my responsibility to encourage you to go there if you like a good burger. I say this not because I'm an advocate of burgers per se, but because when you feel like enjoying a great one, I want you to eat what Harbour Public House serves: real food.

Basically, real food is the same as whole foods, or foods that are made of just one ingredient or are combined only with ingredients we recognize. (I'll talk more about that later in the section So What Should I Eat? An Introduction to Whole Foods, on page 47.) But when it comes to knowing what's okay to eat, we Americans have lost our way. Eating from a food supply that has "advanced" much faster than our bodies have been able to adapt has increased our nation's struggles with heart disease, stroke, type 2 diabetes, cancer, and allergies. These sometimes life-threatening conditions are fairly recent epidemics; they didn't emerge as major health issues until the latter half of the twentieth century. That Morgan Spurlock gained upwards of twenty-four pounds in a month eating mostly burgers at McDonald's, a feat made famous in his 2004 documentary, *Super Size Me*, is horrifying. He showed that eating fast food regularly can undoubtedly cause the problems listed above.

But the burgers themselves didn't cause his weight gain (or the other side effects of his experiment, such as mood swings and sexual dysfunction). It was what was *in* the burgers (and the shakes, fries, and chicken) that mattered. High-fructose corn syrup is the third ingredient in a Big Mac bun. The "cheese" on a Big Mac has sixteen ingredients in it. Chicken McNuggets contain more than thirty ingredients. And while I don't advocate counting a food's ingredients as a general practice, I think it's important to point out that part of what gives so-called bad foods (like hamburgers) a bad reputation—meaning that they can cause weight gain or make a person feel poorly—is that they contain ingredients that aren't what our grandparents' generation would identify as food. Have you ever planted sodium aluminum phosphate in your garden? No? How about ammonium chloride or ethoxylated monoglycerides?

By most accounts, the hamburger was first created in 1900 in New Haven, Connecticut, by Louis Lassen, a Danish immigrant, and became famous at the 1904 St. Louis World's Fair. There have been other claims for its invention, of course, all immaterial for the purpose of this book. The point is this: A hundred years ago, a hamburger was a hunk of real beef served between two pieces of real bread. The grass-fed beef, ground from meat grown without hormones or antibiotics, was cooked and seasoned in the restaurant that sold it; placed between buns made of little more than flour, honey, yeast, and water; and served with garnishes (lettuce, tomatoes, onions) grown on farms tended without pesticides. The hamburger of a

What's in My Milkshake?

The average American consumes more than ten pounds of chemical food additives per year. A typical artificial strawberry flavor, like the kind found in a fast-food chain's strawberry milkshake, contains the following ingredients:

amyl acetate
amyl butyrate
amyl valerate
anethol
anisyl formate
benzyl acetate
benzyl isobutyrate
butyric acid
cinnamyl isobutyrate
cinnamyl valerate
cognac essential oil
diacetyl
dipropyl ketone
ethyl acetate
ethyl amyl ketone
ethyl butyrate
ethyl cinnamate
ethyl heptanoate
ethyl heptylate
ethyl lactate
ethyl methylphenylglycidate
ethyl nitrate
ethyl propionate
ethyl valerate
heliotropin

4-hydroxyphenyl-2-butanone (10 percent solution in alcohol)
a-ionone
isobutyl anthranilate
isobutyl butyrate
lemon essential oil
maltol
4-methylacetophenone
methyl anthranilate
methyl benzoate
methyl cinnamate
methyl heptine carbonate
methyl naphthyl ketone
methyl salicylate
mint essential oil
neroli essential oil
nerolin
neryl isobutyrate
orris butter
phenethyl alcohol
rose
rum ether
g-undecalactone
vanillin
solvent

century ago is not the fast-food hamburger of today. Ditto for Spurlock's shakes, fries, and chicken.

Before we dive into the 100-Year Diet—which means, quite simply, that we should eat the same thing people were eating 100 years ago—let me remind you that I was not able to identify "whole foods" as such until my mid-twenties. I spent so much time with poverty and neglect, my two invisible siblings, that I grew up with even less awareness of what constituted nourishment and health than most Americans. I'm not sure I could have defined "food" at age fifteen; until junior high, I thought microwaves were for drying clothes. As you read, please keep in mind that my goal is not to chastise you for making the wrong choices. (I am in no position to judge anyone on past or present food choices.) My hope is to show you a path forward toward health.

How America Eats

I believe the main culprits behind our society's health problems are the quality of our food and the lifestyle that surrounds it. In order to understand our nationwide weight gain and health loss, we need to take a look at some relatively recent changes in food production.

Since the twentieth century, the Standard American Diet—so uniformly patterned across this vast country that it's known in nutritional circles as the S.A.D., an acronym I think is quite appropriate—has been vastly different from anything our species has ever experienced. After thousands of years of eating mostly whole foods, about a hundred years or so ago, we started stripping out those foods' vitamins, minerals, fiber, and other good stuff. For example, farmers began breeding produce for size and sweetness, effectively decreasing the amount of phytonutrients—the chemical compounds in plants usually responsible for their hefty biological benefits—in our fruits and vegetables. In supermarket products, we replaced nutrients with hydrogenated fats, sugar, and a host of other unhealthy additives and preservatives. (*The American Journal of Clinical Nutrition* estimated in 2004 that Americans get 8 percent of their overall calories from high-fructose corn syrup.) We did this to make life easier; buying a packaged cake mix is usually faster than making it from scratch (and few of us know scratch can actually be faster). But almost every increase in convenience has come at the cost of vital nutrients.

The cultural transition from preparing foods from scratch to buying packaged foods was not a smooth one, either. Even though (or perhaps because) they did most of the cooking, women resisted. Packaged foods didn't taste as good. And deep down, most women knew without being told that packaged foods weren't as healthy or made with as much love. Food manufacturers hired psychologists to teach them how to outwit women's instincts. Over time, industrial foods' marketing campaigns won out, and women born into the prepackaged foods culture accepted them more readily than their mothers had. Fast-food restaurants, which started surfacing in the 1950s and were widely popular by the 1970s, added to the unhealthy mix.

Eating foods that have had their original nutrients replaced by unhealthy fillers is like putting regular fuel in a diesel engine; it doesn't work for long. Eventually, the engine—in our case, the body—breaks down and stops running because it's not getting what it needs to operate. Consider our bones, whose job is to hold up our flesh and muscles. They're made of the calcium and magnesium we get from our food. Today, weak bone health has led to an uptick in long-term bone problems. Even our teeth have suffered; recent generations' jaws have been developing poorly, with weaker, thinner bones, causing a narrowing of the human mouth and a general trend toward the need for braces. (If you look at photos of smiling aboriginal people, you'll notice that they usually have straight teeth.)

The same is true of every part of our bodies. The vitamins in food help us to be happier and have better, more even energy, as well as control hormone levels, which help regulate mood swings and keep us at our body's ideal weight. Other minerals (think iron, zinc, and magnesium) help us so that we don't catch every cold going around, and improve hair and nail strength and shine. A diet depleted of vitamins and minerals (which are found in their most abundant, bioavailable form in whole foods) leads, by definition, to a depleted body. But today, because we eat fewer nutrient-rich foods, we eat fewer nutrients than we ever have.

How the World Eats

Although the S.A.D. has spread to some degree to other Westernized developed–world countries, the cultural habit of obsessing over food, diet, and weight is extremely American. In most cultures, people's food choices are based on what is local and in season, rather than what the latest fad diet is prescribing. Yo-yo dieting and calorie counting are not worldwide phenomena. People outside the United States don't feel ashamed after eating a piece of cake the way we do. And for the most part, cultures that follow traditional diets—even if those diets are relatively limited or traditionally contain a large portion of fats—are thinner and healthier than Americans.

Regions with good eating habits can typically thank food traditions that date back much longer than America itself. In Kenya, for example, the Masai people have lived for hundreds of years on a diet consisting almost entirely of raw cow's blood, raw cow's milk, and beef, with occasional fruit, root, and bark consumption. Even those who are considered overweight within the tribe don't show signs of Western diseases such as diabetes or high blood pressure. Similarly, the Inuit, a people who inhabit the Canadian Arctic and subsist mainly on extremely fatty marine mammals such as whales and seals, have an extremely low cardiac death rate when compared to their southern neighbors. While genetics may play a role in how the Masai and Inuit can handle such a limited diet, they are nourished and grounded by their food culture. It gives them peace, connection, and sustenance. It is a source of fulfillment, not stress. Their philosophy around food is basic and solid, not muddled by confusing messages about what and when and how to eat.

As I began traveling worldwide in my twenties, I witnessed that many cultures, from Europe to Africa, Asia, and South America, ate in much the same way their ancestors had eaten thousands of years before. I watched women prepare the same meals their mothers and grandmothers had prepared, often standing in the same spots, with the same utensils (or lack thereof). In southern India, I ate rice and lentils off banana leaves with my hands, as people have done for thousands of years. We ate slowly and deliberately, instead of quickly, like most do in America. More than anything, I was inspired by how much time people spent preparing and enjoying everyday meals; I hadn't realized how much we *move* when we eat here—in the car, on foot, or while commuting.

In Japan, I learned how to fry tempura the way a son had learned from his father, who had learned it from *his* father. It impacted me not just because I was learning about new foods (and noting a lack of packaged foods that was, at that point, exceptional to me), but also because, for the first time, I was witnessing the generational handing down of a food culture. Having grown up without one of my own, I was not in a position to take the experience for granted. Every time I travel, I borrow traditions to bring home, which, over time, have allowed me to create my own food culture and replace the packaged habits I adopted as a kid.

There is also, of course, the French paradox, which describes the apparent magic by which most of France is capable of eating rich, often fatty foods, drinking copious amounts of wine, and enjoying dessert on a regular basis while maintaining "ideal" (i.e. thin) body weights and optimum heart health. I don't call the French (or the Masai, or the Inuit) miraculous. I call them good eaters with good traditions and good intuition. Moving toward the 100-Year Diet helps my clients escape the mind-numbing cycles of sickness and dieting the S.A.D. helped create.

Back to Basics: Defining the 100-Year Diet

Those of us who have created a rigid, unmanageable, even boring approach to food have probably taken too many (often advertising-related) food messages to heart. We've likely lost touch with many of the simple traditions that surround food in other places—really clear, plain habits such as eating sitting down and celebrating milestones with foods we adore. In America, we're confused, overwhelmed, and inflexible. Because so many of us are desperate to lose weight, we swing rope to rope on whichever "miracle" diet we can grasp first. But perhaps strangely, we typically don't have to look back that far to recognize that our grandmothers and great-grandmothers ate differently. Many of us have grandmothers who made pie. During my childhood, my grandmother often served chipped beef gravy on toast, yet in my own family, we didn't have a real dinner.

Not long ago in America, livestock came from small farms, not feedlots. The milkman delivered fresh raw milk and butter to the milk boxes of city homes. The egg man brought fresh, pastured eggs. Grandma made her chicken soup and kept it on the back of the stove for a week without worrying about bacteria. The word "carbohydrate" wasn't in anyone's vocabulary. Food, at its core, was utterly basic. And people weren't flocking to buy diet books.

I understand that harking back to Grandma's days can present an idealistic view of how America ate just a few generations ago. At the beginning of the twentieth century, life expectancy was fifty years—and people suffered more than we do today from poverty, malnutrition, infectious diseases, and childhood diseases. The point is that, overall, people approached food and nutrition more naturally than we tend to today. They weren't burdened by rules about "good" or "bad" foods or unrealistic expectations about what constitutes a healthy body. When we return to eating real, whole foods, we eliminate the confusion. We re-create a sensible framework on which we can base all our food decisions.

Most of my clients have tried so many diets and have built up so many emotions surrounding food choices—guilt, shame, and unrealistic expectations are most common—that the most important thing I can offer them is a way to eliminate some of the stress that surrounds eating. I don't want you to wake up crying because you're sad and anxious about food and terrified to open the refrigerator every morning. (That's what many of my clients report.) I call it the 100-Year Diet because it's inherently easier to make choices when you think of foods in terms of their existence a century ago. Only, it's not really a specific diet. It's an approach that involves two things:

eating whole foods—the ones you can imagine people eating at the start of the twentieth century—and understanding that food has changed a lot in (relatively) recent history.

So What Should I Eat? An Introduction to Whole Foods

Food is what fuels us. We need it, period. What we don't need is the stress that surrounds choosing it. But for many of us, the process of choosing "healthy" foods has become so fraught and complicated that, in desperation, we often wind up eating packaged foods because it seems easier than figuring out what foods are most nutritious. It seems easier, faster, and cheaper than learning how to cook. For most people, researching a food's nutritional information is akin to taking a drink from a fire hose; you end up getting blasted with more information than you really need. But ultimately, there's only one guideline you need when you choose each meal: eat whole foods.

As Cynthia Lair states, **whole foods are foods that are made of just one ingredient (such as apples, eggs, or beans) or are combined only with whole ingredients we recognize (such as bread made with just whole wheat flour, water, salt, and yeast)**. A whole food is also a food that can be found in nature; it's rich in nutrients that our bodies are able to break down and assimilate into the proteins, carbohydrates, and fats used for energy. Finally, whole foods are usually foods we can imagine growing or being raised in a natural environment.

When we make whole foods the foundation of our diet, we start a journey toward a healthier immune system, an increase in physical and mental energy, a leaner figure, and a stronger digestive tract. With a little training, whole foods become easier to identify. Here's a simple way to judge your produce, for example: If it comes from a farm or the woods, it's probably much more nutrient dense than anything you can buy at the grocery store. If you're at a supermarket, go for foods with no nutrition label (such as fresh produce, meat, and dairy) or with just one or two (easily pronounceable) ingredients on that label. Shop the perimeter of the grocery store.

If you want to practice identifying whole foods, take a walk down a few aisles at your supermarket. Ranch dressing made to be shelf stable has many more unpronounceable ingredients than fresh, refrigerated ranch dressing. Granola made with just oats, nuts, fruit, butter, and maple syrup does far more for your body than a version made with high-fructose corn syrup and partially hydrogenated oils, even if the latter claims to be made with whole grains in giant red letters on the front. In general, the more whole a food, the better it is for our bodies. Orange juice isn't a "bad" food, but whole oranges have more of the natural fiber that is often missing from their juiced counterpart. The same is true for olive oil versus whole olives—eaten whole, olives have better anti-inflammatory and antioxidant benefits than olive oil.

Consider milk, one of the quintessential foods considered healthy but often avoided by dieters in its whole form. Skim milk has fewer calories than whole milk, but it's also missing some of the crucial nutrients found in whole milk—namely, the fat required to maintain bone health. All milk has calcium, which alone can strengthen bones, but bones are only strong *and flexible* when the calcium is consumed with the right combination of magnesium, vitamin D, and essential fatty acids—the proportions found naturally in organic whole milk from healthy animals. Consuming whole milk, instead of skim, gives us the perfect mix, so we don't need to depend on supplements to support bone health. (I know that the idea of switching from skim to full-fat milk makes people panic; I'll explain fat's role in satiety and hormone regulation later in this chapter.)

Many people feel constantly deflated because, while they feel they're making smart choices about what they choose to nibble on, they can't seem to stop snacking and snacking and snacking. From a physiological standpoint, that's totally expected. When we eat a lot of partial foods, which is typically what happens when we eat packaged snack foods, our body craves the parts it doesn't get and tells us to keep eating. (I tend to laugh at those old Pringles commercials. Of course you can't stop eating them—there's nothing in them that tells your body it's getting food!) Choosing whole foods often results in improved health and weight loss simply because our body's innate wisdom tells us to stop eating sooner when we consume the things it actually needs.

Cynthia Lair's Whole Foods Quiz

My friend and colleague Cynthia Lair, a Seattle-based cookbook author who was an early pioneer of the whole foods movement, says that when we come face-to-face with a food in the grocery store, we should ask ourselves the following questions:

- How many ingredients does this food have?
  (If it is a whole food, it has one ingredient, or is a compilation of all recognizable whole foods ingredients.)
- What has been done to it since it was harvested?
  (Hopefully not much.)
- Is this product part of a food or the whole thing?
  (Juice vs. whole fruit.)
- Can I picture this food growing in a field?
  (Apple: yes. Doritos: no, unless you have a great imagination.)

What, Exactly, Are Processed Foods?

A large proportion of the food available today in America no longer resembles anything found in nature. Our food is stripped, refined, bleached, injected, hydrogenated, chemically treated, irradiated, and gassed. Modern foods have longer shelf lives because they've literally had the life taken out of them to preserve them. Highly processed foods have neither the beneficial bacteria (probiotics) nor the food these bacteria require to live (prebiotics) we require for digestive health and nutrient absorption. (If we scour our food history, it's clear that many of our everyday foods a hundred years ago were fermented and loaded with probiotics—think wine, cheese, and hot sauce. I'll explore probiotic foods more in Chapter 4.) With the industrial revolution and the increased need to ship food long distances, such foods fell out of favor because they weren't shelf stable. They were a nuisance for manufacturers.

Another way to define whole foods is to come at it from the back end and learn to identify (and avoid) processed foods. By law, manufacturers are required to list significant ingredients and preservatives on a food's nutrition label. You can tell a food is processed if its ingredients list contains preservatives such as sodium nitrate, sulfites, sodium benzoate, butylated hydroxyanisole, or butylated hydroxytoluene. My guideline is that if I can't pronounce something, or if an ingredients list is miles long, I don't want to eat it regularly. Packaging is another simple clue; if a food comes in a cellophane wrapper or in packaging that obscures the actual product, it has typically been processed.

Beyond preservatives, processed foods also contain additives and chemicals our bodies are unable to recognize. A good example is high-fructose corn syrup (HFCS), which is a sweetener found in many brands of soda and candy—but also in frozen pizza, flavored yogurt, applesauce, ketchup, and other foods we might not always associate with added sweeteners. Because our bodies haven't been genetically designed to break down HFCS, our liver is tasked with trying to eliminate it from our bodies. Years of soda and processed foods consumption bombards and exhausts the liver, which then tells the body to store HFCS and other toxins (like trans fats, refined sugar, and artificial food colorings) in our fat cells instead. Then our immune system kicks in by producing inflammation in an effort to destroy the toxins. Although it can be painful and uncomfortable, it's actually our body's way of trying to protect us by getting rid of foods that are, in effect, invaders. Over time, eating processed foods and their accompanying toxins can cause us to develop inflammatory conditions, digestive disorders, joint degeneration, autoimmune disorders, hyperactivity, and depression.

Behind the Mask

Most dieters, especially lifelong dieters, know that in general, squishy white bread and packaged brownies aren't ideal for the body, while whole foods are. We all know we need vegetables, right? The foods that trick us, though, are the foods masquerading as health foods—things like gluten-free products and frozen dinners, whose ingredient lists often need to be printed in teensy letters because they're so lengthy. Next time you pass through the freezer aisle, try reading the ingredients on a name-brand packaged meal. You may be surprised to learn that some of the foods you've been depending on to lose weight contain huge numbers of unhealthy, unnatural ingredients.

The strange substances found in some of our processed foods can also be detrimental to weight-loss efforts. When our cells take in unknown particles, they get in the way of our body's natural metabolic processes. Cell-to-cell signaling, detoxification, and the release of the hormones that keep our metabolism moving all come to a halt. (Processed non-food products, such as lotions and deodorants, can also have a detrimental effect on our hormonal system. I'll talk about natural alternatives to those in Chapter 9.) Moving away from processed foods—without getting overly rigid—is a crucial step toward health.

Please note, however, that avoiding processed food doesn't mean giving up the foods you love. If you're hungry for beef stroganoff, a version made with grass-fed beef, fresh carrots and celery, real sour cream, and fresh noodles beats the kind you find in a box on the shelf in the pasta aisle. If you always eat pizza on Friday nights, keep doing it—just make it with ingredients your grandmother would have used, like real cheese, tomatoes, and a whole-grain crust.

Keeping it Practical

We don't all have time to make homemade pizza crust every night. I get that. In my household, I'm often feeding five adults (or almost-adults), and I know how hard it can be to land at home after a full day and suddenly be faced with the challenge of preparing something simultaneously healthy and delicious. (I feel grateful every week for the frozen pizza dough my local grocer carries, which is made with the same ingredients I would use if I were making it myself and is sold in a neat little ball, all ready to go.)

Most of us have full-time jobs and families to care for, which leaves less time for cooking. And, truth be told, many of us don't even *like* cooking. In the past, women often spent eight to ten hours a day preparing food—a practice still common in some cultures around the world. They chopped their own vegetables, ground their own spices, and regularly butchered their own meat. In his 2013 book *Cooked*, Michael Pollan reports that Americans are buying more prepared meals every year and cooking less: just twenty-seven minutes per day. We as a culture simply don't value food preparation and cooking. In my twenties, even twenty minutes would have sounded extravagant to me. (Truthfully, I didn't know one could spend that much time cooking. I was that ignorant about food.)

I know many of my clients can't even begin to imagine spending more than a half hour on dinner each night. Others balk at the cost of vegetables like artichokes and asparagus. I tell them this: It's okay. Do the best you can with the amount of time and money you have. And note that, according to Carlo Petrini, founder of the Slow Food movement, in the 1960s Americans spent 18 percent of their budget on food and 5 percent on health care. Today we spend 9 percent on food and 16 percent on health care. It's not *whether* you want to spend the money; it's *where* you want to spend it.

Focusing on whole foods doesn't mean you can never buy canned soup or frozen vegetables or anything that comes in a package ever again. (In fact, research has shown that because they're frozen within hours of picking, frozen vegetables are often just as high or higher in nutrient value than some fresh vegetables. The goal is to get the vegetables in; five servings or more of fruits and vegetables a day are linked to a 46 percent reduction in breast cancer risk, whether they're fresh or frozen.) While it's good to strive for products with ingredients you can pronounce, the point is not to create outrageously high expectations. Going crazy does not make you healthier. If we find ourselves saying we "should" be chopping all our own vegetables, making our own chicken broth from scratch every week, and baking our own bread, we need to take a deep breath and relax.

Our job is to figure out what prepared foods we can't live without and find the brands that are as good for our bodies as possible. Read a product's ingredients and decide whether it's "whole" enough for you on that particular day. This is a great opportunity to move away from all-or-nothing thinking and practice what I call the *Living in the Gray Guideline: Aim for the gray area. Eat the best you can as much as you can. Forget about perfection.* This means that while you may be trying new things every day, you don't have to give up the foods that you may think make life worth living—if you're a die-hard fan of canned, chemically preserved enchilada sauce, fine. (That's what I use to cook for my family, because that's what works for us.)

Marc David, founder of the Institute for the Psychology of Eating and author of *The Slow Down Diet*, advocates a similar philosophy, the 80/20 Guideline, which advocates people eat as well as they can 80 percent of the time. Of course, if they're given numbers, some people may be tempted to count. (Am I at 79 percent for the week yet? Or already to 82 percent?) I'd prefer you didn't. Just be as honest as you can with yourself about aiming for healthy habits without becoming too rigid.

The other reality is that we all have weaknesses. When I'm hungry and there's nothing readily available in the refrigerator, I've been known to have potato chips scooped into sour cream for dinner. I *love* dipping french fries in ranch dressing. Instead of using these eating habits to label ourselves as weak willed or punishing ourselves for succumbing to them, we should embrace them and use them as opportunities to improve how we make food choices. I buy potato chips made with just potatoes, oil, and salt, and pair them with real, full-fat cultured sour cream. Want a milkshake? Instead of hitting the drive-through for a strawberry milkshake made with the ingredients listed on page 41, make your own, with great vanilla ice cream and berries frozen at peak ripeness. Want a burger? Find a good one made with real ingredients.

Food for Thought

While some people associate the term "health food" with fruits and vegetables and the whole foods described in this chapter, others conjure up images of eating only tree bark and steamed lentils. But why does the term exist at all? All food is supposed to be healthy, right?

All Food Has Changed

You know now, if you didn't before, that the packaged cupcake that lists a paragraph's worth of ingredients is a processed food. But our food supply has changed over the centuries in less obvious ways too. Consider meat and poultry. A hundred years ago, beef were raised grazing on open pastureland, and chickens were given free range in grassy areas. These days, most US livestock are raised in cramped quarters on feedlots, fed genetically modified corn and soy, and injected with hormones that cause them to gain body mass more quickly. Chickens are stuffed into crowded cages, where they can't practice their normal behaviors (like, you know, walking). In both cases, these unnatural conditions lead to stress and illnesses, which require antibiotics. Just like us, animals are what they eat. As a result, when we eat grain-fed beef and unhealthy chickens, our bodies have to absorb the hormones and antibiotics that the animals themselves have absorbed, and our health suffers. Following are tips for what to look for when you shop.

Meats

In general, seek out meats that are as natural as possible. Pastured chickens are a better choice than cooped-up chickens. Grass-fed beef is superior to factory-farmed beef because the meat is richer in nutrients and healthy fats. Typically, grass-fed meat will not be labeled "organic" (even though it often meets organic standards) because pastured cows require an enormous amount of land on which to graze, and it is typically cost-prohibitive for ranchers to buy the land (as opposed to leasing it) and go through the process required to earn the label.

If you've walked through a high-end natural grocery store recently, you've likely noted that these choices come with a higher price tag. It's well earned; factory farms' unhealthy practices drastically cut the costs associated with raising meat. Learn to make less expensive choices for your family. Steak is reserved for special occasions at my house, whereas roasts and stew meat are more common. I buy whole chickens because they're less expensive. When we purchase healthy meats, we are doing something better for our bodies, but also voting against the unhealthy practices of feedlot farming.

Salt

For millennia, humans have used salt as a preservative, a flavoring agent, and as currency. (The word "salary" is derived from the Latin *salarium*, which was the money paid to Roman soldiers for their regular purchase of salt.) Anthropologists have found evidence of salt currency in sub-Saharan Africa, salt offerings in Egyptian tombs, and salt mines in China dating to 6000 BC. It played an important role in India's emancipation from British rule. But in the last century, salt's role has evolved from essential to taboo.

Modern research has failed to link salt consumption to increased cardiovascular disease or a shorter lifespan. Most studies—including a seminal 1970s experiment that fed rats about sixty times as much salt as the average human consumes and reported it to be dangerous—are incomplete at best. Interestingly, evidence from recent studies has shown just the opposite:

failing to incorporate salt into our diets can actually cause premature death. Our bodies use salt to regulate fluid balance, control muscle contractions, balance adrenal and thyroid glands, and guide nerve impulses. I approach salt with common sense; it's clear that most animals like it (think of the salt licks farmers put out for their livestock) and human athletes require extra when they work hard, so it stands to reason that the rest of us, as long as we have healthy kidneys that can process it, need it also.

Note, though, that "salt" means more than one thing. Gary Taubes, *Why We Get Fat* author and pro-salt advocate, reminded readers in *Science* magazine that 80 percent of the salt Americans get is from processed foods. In those cases, salt is used as a preservative and flavor enhancer—jobs it's done well throughout history. But today, processed food producers rely on iodized salt (also known as table salt), which is mined, chemically refined, and often blended with anticaking agents to make it free flowing. (The government began regulating salt additives in the early part of the twentieth century. Iodine helps prevent hypothyroidism; it was added to salt because most people don't eat enough seaweed and fish, both natural sources of iodine, in their regular diet.)

Iodized salt does a great job of keeping foods shelf stable, but it doesn't contain the mineral components required for the body's basic functions—note that studies on hypertension, once connected to high salt intake, are typically done on patients consuming only iodized salt, which creates an imbalance in the body when consumed without sea salt's natural minerals. Fine-grain sea salt, which comes from the ocean, is what I prefer. It contains the full complement of minerals available in seawater—including magnesium, calcium, potassium, some iodine, and traces of algae—which, not coincidentally, almost exactly mimics the mineral makeup of human blood. Use sea salt to flavor your food, and use plenty of it. Note too that not all sea salt is created equally. If it's pure white, it has likely been refined. Minerals have color, so true high-quality, mineral-rich sea salt will have pink, brown, and other colored flecks in it. Use salt that looks like it has a little personality.

Dining Out

Food tastes better at great restaurants because they use real fat, high-quality pastured animal meats (usually highlighted on the menu), house-made breads, and plenty of salt in the kitchen. In most ways, this means it's totally fine, from a nutritional standpoint, to eat at restaurants as often as you'd like. However, the restaurants that serve excellent food are usually more expensive; cheaper restaurants keep costs down by using packaged, shelf-stable foods, factory-farmed meats and dairy, and lower-quality vegetables. If you can afford to eat at high-end restaurants often, great—but not everyone can. So if we're not eating whole foods when we dine out, we should revert to the habits we had a century years ago, and save restaurants for special occasions.

Milk

In the last century, the dairy industry has undergone changes similar to those in the meat industry. Like us, cows are what they eat. Instead of grazing on grass, many conventional dairy cows feed mostly on corn and soy, which means they don't make milk rich in the vitamins and minerals found in grassy open pastureland. Among other things, organic labeling regulations require livestock be allowed to graze. (There are some organic brands that do not follow these guidelines, which often leads co-ops to refuse to carry their products. Learn to ask questions at the market.) Choosing organic milk and dairy products over conventional ones ensures, at least in part, that some of what fills your glass came from the kinds of grasses and shrubs cows want to munch on naturally.

A nationwide 2013 Washington State University study showed that, when averaged over a year, organic milk had 62 percent more omega-3 fatty acids (the kind that reduce inflammation and help our skin and brain) than conventional milk. Consuming organic over conventional would, researchers said, reduce or eliminate probable risk factors for a wide range of developmental and chronic health problems.

The Health Benefits of Grass-Fed Products

- **Better-quality fat:** Grass-fed meat naturally contains up to a third less fat than feedlot beef, which can translate to weight loss (see page 245, Answer #10 in Quiz).
- **Omega-3s:** Meat from grass-fed animals has two to four times more omega-3 fatty acids, which are known to help prevent heart disease and decrease inflammation, than meat from grain-fed animals.
- **CLA:** Meat and dairy products from grass-fed ruminants are the richest known source of a "good" type of fat called conjugated linoleic acid, or CLA, which increases the rate at which we burn fat and helps prevent cancer.
- **Vitamin E:** Meat from pastured cattle is four times higher in vitamin E, which is great for our skin and cardiovascular health, than the meat from feedlot cattle.

Importantly, though, I recommend my clients drink whole milk. Americans have been conditioned to believe only children need full-fat milk to support their developing brains, ignoring the fact that adults, too, need whole milk's saturated fats. The main vitamins milk is known to impart, vitamins A and D, are fat soluble, which means that when consumed in the absence of fat, we don't absorb them. While skim or low-fat milk does indeed contain fewer calories than whole milk, the latter has more health benefits; the same WSU research reported whole milk was upwards of 50 percent higher in omega-3s than low-fat or skim milks. Whole milk also offers satiety, so those who partake often feel fuller, faster. (Now is probably the time to tell you I drink heavy cream by the glass, especially during the winter months, because I feel that's what my body needs.)

Eggs

You've seen the woman standing with glazed eyes at the grocery store's egg case. She picks up one carton, then another, inspecting their contents not just for broken shells but perhaps also for some sort of omen to show her whether cage-free, organic, free-range, or just plain eggs are best for her family. Maybe that woman was you.

I hate to be a Debbie Downer, but that woman was buying eggs in the wrong place. Although the look and content of an egg hasn't changed much in a hundred years—they're much cleaner today, I suppose, and now need to be refrigerated in the United States because the protective coating they come with naturally, called the bloom, is usually washed off here—their nutritional value has plummeted because chickens no longer eat real chicken food.

Next time you're standing in the egg aisle, buy a carton of your usual eggs. Then, go to a farmers' market and buy eggs from a farmer who says his chickens scratch and dig and eat bugs, which is what chickens have evolved to do. Crack one of each egg into a white bowl, and look at the difference in color. The yolk of the grocery store egg—even a cage-free one—will be lighter in color and sort of defeated-looking, while the vibrant, orange-hued farm egg will be buoyant and round because it has more of the nutrients that make eggs the ideal food. The egg is healthier because the chicken is healthier. Then cook the eggs separately: you'll notice that the more nutritious egg tastes a lot better too. When you can, buy eggs that come from pastured chickens that can act like chickens.

Produce

The Chinese are famous for saying Westerners have to take bitter pills because they don't eat bitter foods. We can't deny it; a trip through an Asian grocery store makes it clear that while most Western vegetables are prized for their sweetness and size, Eastern equivalents are often valued for bitterness and bite. (For fun, compare American and Asian varieties of eggplants, cucumbers, leafy greens, and pears. The downside, for

Americans, is that the bitter or astringent taste in many vegetables is caused by phytonutrients, the very things our bodies need.

We like our vegetables sweet because we've been well trained, both by nature and by industry. Since the advent of agriculture, humans have picked the sweetest crops to promulgate, growing plants high in sugars and thus, carbohydrates, because they were tastier to eat. But in the last century, with the advancements of American agricultural science, the trend has turned many of our fruits and vegetables into candy as compared to their historical counterparts. It's as simple as fruit salad: the most popular American varieties of apples and grapes, for example, are sweeter than their European cousins and much less nutritious.

While many cultures regularly consume dandelion greens, a "superfood" that the *New York Times* reported in 2013 to have seven times the phytonutrients of spinach, we as a country often look down on wild foods (or nonmainstream foods) as somehow less acceptable than what we find in the supermarket. That, or we label foods that haven't been exposed to scientific toying as "miracles" because they actually contain the vitamins and minerals our bodies crave. But many of these so-called miracle foods, such as seaweeds, wild greens, organ meats, fermented foods, and shellfish (which I discuss in Chapter 7) are often miraculous simply because they haven't been messed with. The nutrition hasn't been bred out of them.

When you shop, look for vegetables with a lot of color, which is often a sign of how healthy a food can be for you. Pick yellow corn over white, dark purple or red carrots over orange, potatoes with colored flesh over those with white interiors. Choose darker lettuces over light. Branch out, encouraging yourself to try a new vegetable every now and then, including herbs, which historically haven't been tampered with much. Also, aim for green vegetables such as broccoli, because that green color is actually masking all sorts of colors underneath. Eating more green vegetables means you are actually eating a rainbow of color (read: nutrients) in each bite. At the grocery store, I buy organic dairy and meats (especially beef) whenever possible. (Because cows are such big animals, and require so much feed, their bodies accumulate higher levels of toxins as they grow as compared to smaller animals, like chickens. All that gets passed on to us.) I consider organic vegetables ideal but optional; I buy them when they are affordable and in season.

The Oxygen Mask Rule

We've all heard flight attendants instruct us before an airline flight to secure our own oxygen mask before assisting others. The same is true with food. As girlfriends, spouses, moms, and caring hostesses, many women practice great eating habits but constantly put others—often children and partners—before themselves, sometimes going as far as buying better ingredients for their children than they do for themselves. Put on your own mask first.

Bread

I don't bake my own bread, and I certainly don't remember my mother or grandmother baking bread. But in this case, my own history isn't much different from many others'. In contrast to my teenage years, when a bite of a friend's sandwich invariably consisted of snowy-white bread, I now typically eat artisanal sourdough bread or bread made with sprouted grains.

But the way we define bread has changed. A hundred years ago, bread was usually fermented, meaning it had undergone a long rising process, often involving natural bacteria that break down the proteins and yeast in the loaf, making the gluten much easier to digest. (Many people who feel they're sensitive to gluten find they're fine with fermented breads or anything made with a sourdough starter, because the fermentation process is in essence a predigesting process.) Bread was designated as "fresh" because over the course of a day or two, it went stale.

Today, "bread" often means packaged presliced loaves; even the whole-grainiest types last for a week or two on the counter without losing their squish and moisture. We've grown to value convenience over flavor and wholesomeness. As a result, the insides of our loaves have changed. Instead of five or six ingredients, many types of bread have upwards of twenty. Most shelf-stable products now have a higher gluten content, making breads more difficult to digest; gluten creates predictability in baked goods and allows for easier (read: more cost-efficient) mechanized dough handling.

When you buy bread, make sure you're buying *bread*. Read the ingredients—or better yet, buy it directly from a baker who can tell you what went into it without pausing for a breath.

Power Versus Poison

The beauty of food in the twenty-first century is that we have options. Restaurants, grocery stores, farmers' markets, and co-ops around the country offer huge varieties of whole foods. Rather than buying foods that effectively poison us—redefining "food poisoning" is on my to-do list—we should focus on foods we can, as Cynthia Lair says, imagine growing in a field or hanging on a branch. Eating whole foods does not require building backyard chicken coops, learning to grind wheat berries for flour, or using every grain in the bulk section. The goal here is not perfection. The goals are realism and intention.

....

THE PRESCRIPTION

- Eat whole foods, including real meat, dairy, eggs, produce, high-quality sea salt, and bread, that have been processed as minimally as possible.
- At the grocery store, read the list of ingredients on the products you commonly buy. Look for minimal lists with ingredients you can pronounce.
- Follow the Living in the Gray Guideline (see page 53); eating whole foods means doing so in as practical a way as possible.
- Choose thoughtful restaurants. Eat at spots that list grass-fed beef, local produce, and dairy they're proud of on the menu.

Chapter 4

A GUT FEELING

You aren't what you eat. You're what you absorb.

—Nutritionists' adage

You know the symptoms of poor digestion: bloating, nausea, gas, belching, and diarrhea. Even those with the strongest stomachs have had them. In my early twenties, when my peers were partying, I was imprisoned by my digestive tract. I staged every social engagement with an escape plan, so I could run home to use the bathroom or lie down to ease the pain while my stomach swelled up as if I were five months pregnant. I farted like a frat boy, so I lived like a monk. While my girlfriends organized dates, I was visiting doctors, dropping off stool samples, and filling prescription after prescription for antibiotics that never worked for long. Many of the professionals I saw advised me to restrict my diet. Doctors prescribed pharmaceuticals, and holistic practitioners prescribed supplements, but both sides apologetically agreed that I would probably never be able to eat many everyday foods.

I spent *so* much time on my bed in the fetal position. I got to know my knees very, very well, all the time rationalizing that, if the doctors couldn't explain them, my symptoms must be an outer expression of some deeper, inner flaw. They matched what I had always suspected about myself: that I *was* different, somehow tainted. I assumed that if anyone knew the truth about me—about my history or about my digestion—they would run for the hills. I became even more ashamed of my body. Dating was out of the question.

What I know now, after years of study and research, is that I *was* different. A lifetime of malnutrition, scavenging, and the heavy-metal toxicity so common in most of our bodies, coupled with my parasite exposure in South America, had taken its toll on my digestive system. Decades of neglect had left me with irritable bowel syndrome, chronic fatigue, multiple food sensitivities, hypothyroidism, anemia, high cholesterol, and an adrenal system so shot I still marvel that I was able to get out of bed at all. Rebuilding my digestive system from the ground up transformed the way I felt, and, in fact, the way I lived. Understanding that my digestive difficulty wasn't my fault—that it wasn't some kind of karmic mark on my character—would take a whole lot longer.

What's Happening Inside

When our digestive system is working correctly, things seem straightforward: Food goes in; energy and waste come out. We're machines. We work as long as we eat on a regular basis, right?

It's not quite that simple. The human digestive system—a network of millions of neurotransmitters and microbes so intelligent it's often referred to as the body's "second brain"—plays a major role in controlling our physical and emotional state, energy levels, and appetites. From the moment a person sees or smells something tasty, the digestive process begins. The mouth waters. When food touches the tongue, the digestive tract kicks into gear. First, the mouth produces more saliva, which helps break down food.

The esophagus pushes the food into the stomach, where gastric juices rich in enzymes produced by the cells of the stomach lining go to town breaking down the food further. Eventually, the bite of food makes its way into the small intestine, where enzymes, acids, and millions—really, *millions*—of gut microbes break the food down into nutrients that then get absorbed into the bloodstream. It's those tiny bacteria that are ultimately responsible for our overall health, because they're the gatekeepers (and in some cases, the producers) of the nutrients we require for survival. The food then moves to the large intestine, which processes leftover waste and water before it leaves the body.

But poor eating habits, born from a food culture built on marketing and convenience and largely devoid of bacteria, have led to less than stellar digestion for millions of us. As a result, the average American takes in only a fraction of the nutrients in the food he or she eats. You know that old adage, "You are what you eat"? It's not quite so simple. **You are what you digest and absorb.** You can have the best diet on the planet, but if your body can't manage to properly break down what goes in, your health will suffer—whether you're eating salad or Skittles. (Note that not absorbing nutrients isn't the same thing as not processing calories; there's a common misconception that absorbing more is the same as gaining weight. In fact, as I'll discuss in Chapter 6, an increase in bacteria is what actually causes weight loss for many people, because the bacteria teach the body how to process food properly.)

The Hidden Culprit

Even if you don't experience the more dramatic digestive issues that plagued me, understanding the important role digestion plays in the body is crucial. Digestion is the foundation of health. Our body is made up of the food we eat; if we can't break down our food and extract its nutrients, the body doesn't have the building blocks it needs to heal and repair our cells. As a result, we experience nutritional deficiencies—often exemplified by outward physical

What You Can Learn from Poop

Stools are an extremely convenient way for nutritionists to learn about what's going on in a client's body. Below is a rough list of what I look for, given how clients describe their poop.

- **Black, tarry, sticky:** Can mean bleeding in the upper digestive tract or iron supplementation
- **Very dark brown:** Drank red wine or diet has too much salt or not enough vegetables
- **Glowing red, magenta:** Eaten beets
- **Light green:** Too much sugar, too many fruits and vegetables with not enough grains and salt
- **Pale or clay colored:** Minimal amounts of bile being excreted, gallbladder or liver issues
- **Bloody or mucus covered:** Hemorrhoids, overgrowth of bacteria in gastrointestinal tract, colitis, Crohn's disease, colon cancer, issue near the end of the digestive tract
- **Pencil thin, ribbonlike:** Polyp may be narrowing the passageway, spastic colon
- **Floating, large with greasy film on the toilet water:** Malabsorption
- **Loose, watery with undigested food:** Food poisoning, food allergies, antibiotics, antacids, dietary changes, travel, anxiety, stress, irritable bowel syndrome
- **Small, hard, round pellets:** Constipation, too much dry food, laxative abuse, worries, irritable bowel syndrome, not enough vegetables
- **Alternating bouts of constipation and diarrhea:** Irritable bowel syndrome, food allergies, irregular hours, chaotic relationships
- **Foul smell:** Imbalance of intestinal bacteria, too much animal protein
- **Healthy stool:** Smooth, soft, and formed like a banana

signs such as weak, ridged fingernails; brittle hair; dull skin; and vacant eyes. But poor digestion leads to internal symptoms too. If we can't transform food into energy properly, for example, we feel tired. If we feel tired, we usually eat more sugar. If we eat more sugar, we typically gain weight.

That the gut contributes to more than just the digestive process is an important tenet for most doctors. Any good medical practitioner—whether mainstream, holistic, or Eastern—will check a patient's digestion, even for symptoms not commonly thought of as being rooted in the gut, such as extra weight, low energy, skin rashes, or bad breath. (You may remember how, in the movie *The Last Emperor*, a physician checks the boy king's stools to determine whether he is healthy; it's common for Chinese medicine practitioners to examine stools for evidence of digestive health.) In most Western practices, even if doctors do check what's coming *out*, they don't often consider what goes *in*. At Passionate Nutrition, I take a huge departure from America's conventional wisdom. It's all one tube. I link the choices we make on the front end with the problems we face on the back end. And more often than not, I solve those problems for my clients.

Perhaps most importantly, poor digestion is often the source of depression and anxiety. Dr. Michael Gershon, a leading researcher in the field of neurogastroenterology and the author of *The Second Brain*, which reveals the science behind the brain-gut connection, suggests the gut impacts our emotional state in profound ways. As Gershon explains, the gut boasts a whopping 100 million neurons, all intricately folded throughout the digestive tract. (That's more than in any other part of the body outside the brain, including the spinal cord.) Through these neurons, the gut sends signals to the brain to produce a feeling. An unhappy gut sends impulses that produce feelings of stress and sadness—feelings that negatively influence decision making, learning, and even memory. His research shows that how we treat our digestive system directly affects how we feel. People with happy guts are happier and often eat less overall. In other words, the secret to happiness is often good digestion. And as a plus, good digestion may encourage weight loss.

The moment I started paying attention to my gut, my entire life changed. I felt better, I looked better, and I was truly happier. I am no longer confined by the limited diet that I thought was my life sentence; I am now able to eat almost anything.

At my practice, many clients walk in hoping to achieve weight loss by a certain date, say an upcoming birthday or social event—something that may be possible in some cases. The problem is that if a nutritionist treats only the immediate symptoms and prescribes a very limited diet, their client may lose weight, but they can't stick to that diet, and the resulting rebound weight gain is even harder to lose. Further, the underlying causes of being overweight remain completely ignored. In our culture, the first reaction we all (but especially woman) have is to blame ourselves for our problems, including health problems. Like I did, we presume that addressing our (fill in the blank: anxiety, depression, weight issues, digestive stress) would be easy if we were stronger, had more willpower, or were generally better people. We fault ourselves for our discomforts. Meanwhile, we totally ignore how much the food we eat affects how we feel.

That gut health is a crucial key to weight loss comes as a surprise to most of my clients, but over and over, I've watched them lose weight before we even begin addressing things such as sugar cravings (see Chapter 5) and listening to the body's hunger signals (see Chapter 8). I take the long-term approach, tackling every client's digestive health first as a matter of course, because improving digestion remedies issues I wasn't initially called in to address, such as skin problems or bloating, and tends to improve overall health, including mental health. That's why many psychiatrists, psychologists, and therapists send me referrals; they've found that dietary changes make a difference in their clients' emotional well-being and can decrease the amount of medication needed. But even with weight loss as the primary goal, gut health must come first. Digestion is just that powerful.

Five Goals for a Good Gut

Given the myriad ways we can screw up our digestive system, it's only fair that, in turn, we can rely on a number of tried-and-true methods for repairing it. I start on the path to healthy digestion by adding foods that heal. For those with severe digestive issues or painful gut inflammation, this usually means starting slowly, showing clients how gentle foods (foods that are easy to digest) can calm abdominal pain and improve energy, among other things. I add nourishing, mineral-dense bone broth to heal the lining of the gut (see page 241 for a recipe). I teach people to embrace bacteria and explain both their role in the body and in the digestive process. Then I introduce fermented foods that establish a healthy balance of those good bacteria within our digestive tracts. Finally, I talk about *how* we eat, giving clients actionable tactics for eating mindfully and learning to listen to their bodies.

Note that the following suggestions are listed in the order in which you should incorporate them into your diet; you don't have to do them all at once at first. As always, because change is difficult, you don't have to take a black-and-white approach. Follow the Living in the Gray Guideline (see page 53). Also know that the recommendations that follow regarding cutting foods out are not meant to be lifelong sentences. If your digestive system is especially weak, you may need to cut back on troublesome foods like raw vegetables at first, but many of us can reintroduce the foods that bother us once our system is strong again. (This does not, however, apply to certain conditions, such as severe food allergies or celiac disease.)

Gut Goal #1: Eat Gentle Foods

You know how passionately I believe in the power of whole foods. However, if the digestive tract isn't strong enough to digest a whole food—say, brown rice or a raw carrot—eating it can do us more harm than good. It can bring back the pain we wanted to relieve in the first place. Many clients come in after switching from a highly processed diet to eating "healthier" foods such as raw salads and whole-grain breads. They come to me frustrated and in pain because their digestive systems can't handle things such as quinoa, beans, and raw kale. They want to go back to name-brand boxed meals because it doesn't hurt; I don't blame them. I had the same thing happen. Bloating and cramping after eating raw vegetables, whole-grain breads, and legumes is a sign that your gut needs a good dose of R&R, in the form of soft, overcooked, low-fiber foods. If whole foods hurt, your gut needs some time to heal.

When clients come to me with severe digestive issues, such as ulcerative colitis, Crohn's disease, debilitating gas and bloating, or severe hemorrhoids, I often prescribe such a diet. Most report that when they complained to their traditional doctors about pain, the doctors encourage higher fiber intake. Fiber is one of the harshest things a person can consume—it's known as "nature's scrub brush" for a reason. I recommend the tender loving care that comes in the form of easily digestible foods. Anything soft, moist, and very cooked will do the trick; the more you cook a food, the less work your body has to do to digest it. (You can think of raw food proteins as balls of yarn wrapped around nutrients; the body has to unravel the yarn before it can use what's in the center. Cooking the proteins does half the unraveling for you, so your stomach has less work to do and actually gets to the nutritious stuff in the middle.) For many clients, go-tos include slow-cooked meat, custard, applesauce, winter squash, yams, sweet potatoes, and pâté. You can eat what you want—including highly flavored foods—as long as you avoid very fibrous foods and can cut all of your food with a fork.

Eating soft foods can also help combat fatigue. The less energy your body spends digesting foods, the more it saves for daily activities. Most of my clients are amazed by how quickly this approach helps; within days or weeks, their bodies begin absorbing nutrients more effectively, and they see a notable decrease in pain and increase in energy.

The biggest barrier to eating gentle foods is usually the brain. Even though soft stuff might be good for our particular condition, we're simply not good at eating anything that mimics baby food. As adults, we feel entitled to eat crunchy, chewy, fibrous foods. But something akin to baby food might be just what we need. (In fact, I advocate that clients with severe digestive issues eat jarred baby food if they don't feel like they have the time or energy to cook foods properly.)

Soft Foods for an Inflamed Gut

The following foods, cooked until they can be cut with a fork, can be easy to digest:

Proteins
- Beef roasts, slow-cooked
- Chicken, slow-cooked
- Eggs
- Salmon or low-mercury tuna
- Broth soups
- Pâté
- Soft white fish (like cod or halibut)

Grains
- White rice
- White sourdough bread (cold or toasted)
- Congee
- Rice pudding

Vegetables
- Winter squash
- Root vegetables
- Avocados (raw is okay)

Fruit
- Applesauce
- Cooked fruit compote
- Baked apples
- Baked pears

Fats
- Coconut milk
- Coconut oil
- Butter (raw or cold is okay)

We also get so caught up in what other people say is healthy that we forget to listen to our own bodies' wisdom. If we know, for example, that we feel okay when we eat white bread but experience agonizing cramps when we eat whole-wheat bread, we shouldn't eat whole-wheat bread, no matter how many times we've heard about its nutritional superiority. Whole-wheat bread isn't better for *you* if your body can't digest it. I know it goes against our current culture, but there are some foods we also get more nutrition from when they are well cooked—asparagus, carrots, tomatoes, and dark-green leafy vegetables such as kale all contain nutrients that are more bioavailable when the vegetables are cooked. (We eat carrots thinking we are getting their beta-carotene, but we are only able to break down and absorb about 3 percent of their beta-carotene when they are raw.) Not everyone needs to eat a diet made up entirely of gentle foods, but if you experience pain or gas and bloating, don't let your mind take over. Try eating gentle foods for three days and see what happens.

You don't need to eat gentle foods forever; eat them for as long as it takes your body to heal. When you feel comfortable eating all gentle foods, begin introducing other foods one at a time—raw soft lettuces, such as butter lettuce, are a good place to start.

Raw or Cooked?

If you have severe digestive issues, raw food can often be too much to tolerate. I frequently see clients racked by pain who want to know why their raw diet is causing them so much misery. Although such diets are all the rage in celebrity circles, handling raw food requires a rock-solid digestive system, which is why Traditional Chinese Medicine and Ayurvedic medicine, the oldest forms of medicine in the world, are based predominantly on cooked foods.

Westerners can use the same approach, but we sometimes require a more scientific explanation. In healthy guts, digestive, metabolic, and food enzymes act as catalysts to help break down and digest food and help support the immune system. But not everyone starts with healthy digestion. Aging, stress, processed foods, and antibiotics and other drugs can inhibit the body's natural enzyme-production process. When the body doesn't have the natural digestive enzyme populations needed to break down food, it can't get through the tough cell walls of foods like plants and tough meats. Cooking these foods slowly, over long periods of time, effectively predigests the cell walls of our food, making its vitamins and minerals easier to absorb and giving our gut a chance to rest and recover. For this reason, even in healthy people, cooked vegetables and fruits, grains, and beans can often provide more nutrients than raw ones.

Gut Goal #2: Drink Bone Broth

Whether you call it chicken soup, beef bouillon, or Jewish penicillin, bone broth has long been known as a remedy for colds and flus because it is one of the world's most healing foods. Made by simmering meat and bones in water with aromatics, it's extremely nourishing, mineral dense, and easy to absorb. Bone broth also helps heal the digestive tract's smooth tissue when it's inflamed, which is the case with many of my clients. I prescribe it for that reason, especially in people with chronic digestive problems, but I also advocate drinking a few cups each day for its "side effects." Bone broth is extremely rich in protein, calcium, and collagen—the same ingredients that make up human bones—so it improves bones, hair, and skin, making them stronger and more resilient. In fact, one of my clients drank bone broth in preparation for, and after, a serious foot surgery, and her doctors were floored by how fast she healed.

Homemade bone broth also makes everyday foods infinitely tastier. When I worked at The Little Nell in Aspen, Colorado, we had bone broth simmering in huge vats; the same is true in most restaurants. Chefs typically add it to dishes, sauces, and stews instead of water because it imparts a deep, rich flavor. At home, I cook my rice in it, use it for all my soups, and drink it plain or seasoned with sea salt, *ume* plum vinegar, or apple cider vinegar. I recommend drinking one to three cups a day (most of the time) to help digestion, strengthen hair, and increase the skin's elasticity. (You'll find a recipe for Bone Broth on page 241.)

Gut Goal #3: Embrace Microbes

There's heavy debate in some homes about whether a dropped morsel of food can stay on the floor for five seconds or thirty. Me? I don't even go by the thirty-second rule, because I'm anti-sterility. Despite a lifetime of watching cleaning commercials, I believe that if we were to completely sterilize our environments, both inside and out, we would die. The bacteria we work so hard to avoid affect almost all of our bodily processes, from weight control to brain health to digestion.

And, well, there are a lot of them, so we should probably play nice. The American Society for Microbiology estimates that the human body is host to ten times more bacteria than human cells—far more than the number of people living on the planet, although the actual figure, estimated to be between 10^{13} (ten trillion), very conservatively, and 10^{14} (a hundred trillion), is debatable. The Human Microbiome Project, a joint research undertaking among about 200 scientists, is mapping the genes of nonhuman organisms hosted by the human body and estimates that the number of different bacteria types involved exceeds 500 (and counting).

E. coli, the bacteria so many of us fear, is just one of those—and as fermentation expert Sandor Ellix Katz reminds us in his book *Wild Fermentation*, the number of "good" bacteria in our bodies far exceeds the number of pathogens. It's those good bacteria that snuggle into the folds and crevices of our gut, making themselves at home so pathogens—the "bad" bacteria—can't find space to live. And while we're born with a certain set of genetic information, those good bacteria—what some call our "second genome"—are malleable and shapeable. As their host, we can help support them, which in turn has an impact on our own genes. However, they do hold the balance of power. That we can pretend to eliminate or control them completely is a human (and very Western) illusion.

In fact, as adults, we've worked hard to introduce bacteria to our bodies. When we're born, our guts are virtually sterile. When we make our way into the world, most typically through the birth canal, we collect our mother's bacteria, which give us our first tools for fighting infection. Studies show that infants born by C-section often have a harder time fighting infection, likely because they aren't inoculated with good pathogen-fighting bacteria during the birth process. As we grow, we move from milk to soft foods to solid foods, collecting along the way all the organisms that live with and in those things. It's no accident that a toddler's stools resemble adult feces; around age three, the bacterial makeup of a child's gut often resembles that of an adult's, as does his or her diet. So baby poop is baby poop because babies haven't amassed the kind of bacteria that make their systems stable (and formula-fed babies tend to have grosser diapers because they're not getting the natural bacteria found in breast milk).

The "good" bacteria—things like *lactobacillus plantarum* and *bifidobacteria*—are the VIPs of the digestive process. They help us digest food, aid in nutrient absorption, produce key vitamins, prevent disease, and much, much more. Scientists recognize that a lack of such good bacteria, a result of living in too-clean environments and eating too-clean foods, may be responsible for the current uptick in autoimmune diseases. But how?

Imagine, if you will, how big an area your skin might cover if you doffed it and spread it out on your dining room table. Inside your gut, the twisty, turny epithelial layer that forms the internal "skin" of your digestive tract is orders of magnitude larger. Many anatomy and physiology courses compare its spread-out size to that of a tennis court, which is an image that always sticks with me. Over every centimeter of that space, the epithelial layer depends for nourishment not on blood, as other body tissues do, but on vitamins and minerals created by the bacteria that line it. The bacteria and their by-products effectively form a protective layer over every inch of that tennis court.

Without a healthy epithelial lining, the gut becomes perforated, allowing toxins and (relatively) large undigested proteins to pass into the bloodstream, rather than being eliminated or broken down. As the bloodstream is filled with these bits the body sees as intruders, the body begins fighting itself, inflammation ensues, and immune issues and food sensitivities are born. The "hygiene hypothesis," a theory that has gained interest in recent years, cites that our changing microbial environment (and the associated decrease in internal bacteria) may be responsible for a whole range of modern chronic ailments, from allergies and inflammatory bowel disease to depression and anxiety.

For years, I've been touting the benefits of good bacteria, and I've noted that clients with healthy bacterial levels are often leaner than those without. Recently, scientists have published a well-defined link between healthy gut bacteria populations and good metabolism. In a 2013 study conducted at

Massachusetts General Hospital, researchers swapped the intestinal bacteria populations of overweight mice and healthy-weight mice but maintained similar diets for each. Not surprisingly, the overweight mice lost weight, while the previously healthy-weight mice gained it. Although the exact method isn't yet known, it's become clear that healthy microbial gut populations have a strong role in regulating metabolism.

Antibiotics, by contrast, which are consumed not just in prescription form but as a by-product of treated meats and dairy, can compromise the body's bacterial balance, as can consuming fluoridated and chlorinated water, processed foods, or high levels of coffee or alcohol. Our job, as eaters, is to keep our gut microbes in balance by constantly replenishing our body's good bacteria. So go ahead, drop something on the floor. Then eat it. I dare you. But more importantly, I suggest you eat the foods that follow.

Gut Goal #4: Introduce Fermented Foods

First, let's cover the basics: Fermentation is the natural process by which microbes such as bacteria and yeast convert sugars, such as those found in fruits and vegetables, into acids, gases, and (in some cases) alcohol. Fermentation occurs naturally inside the gut when the bacteria present there consume prebiotics, which are food *for* bacteria to eat, but eating probiotics, or foods that actually *contain* those bacteria, encourages our guts to act as hosts to good bacteria on a consistent, long-term basis.

Before the advent of refrigeration—actually, before the advent of agriculture—fermented foods played a vital role in the human diet because fermentation was the only means we had for preserving food long term. From bread, cheese, and wine to condiments, pickles, and even soda, which was traditionally a fermented drink served as a digestive tonic, most of the whole foods we eat today can be traced to their fermented ancestors. Yet today, most people eat foods containing live bacteria in miniscule amounts, and then only accidentally. Bread is made with sanitized (nonwild) yeasts, cheese is made with pasteurized milk, and pickles are often bottled and cooked to kill bacteria. When we eat these foods, we eat the products of the fermentation process, but don't enjoy the benefits of the live bacteria themselves.

Finding the Right Fermented Foods

Harvesting the benefits of fermented foods means choosing the right ones and treating them well. When you eat fermented foods, keep the following in mind:

• Look for miso, kimchi, and sauerkraut in the refrigerated section of your supermarket. The products in the unrefrigerated sections have been pasteurized, which means that their beneficial bacteria have been killed. The label should say "raw" or "unpasteurized." You can leave these products on the counter at home if you wish; they will continue to ferment.

• Heating fermented foods kills the beneficial bacteria. Add fermented ingredients to your food after you remove the rest of the meal from the stove or after things like soups and stews have cooled enough for you to stick your finger into them comfortably.

Today, I eat fermented foods at least once a day (most of the time). At home, I ferment everything from cabbage and carrots to milk and mashed potatoes, but because most people don't geek out on fermentation like I do, starting with store-bought fermented foods is the best and easiest way to introduce the body to bountiful levels of good bacteria.

The five probiotic foods I recommend eating—which we call the "Fab Five" at Passionate Nutrition—are kefir, miso, kimchi, various krauts (such as sauerkraut), and apple cider vinegar. At the beginning, I recommend building up your body's reserve of friendly flora by eating two fermented foods a day, in small amounts. Treat fermented foods as condiments you use to flavor a meal, rather than as main courses. Keep in mind that it's normal to experience a bit more gas and bloating right after you start eating fermented foods. You're introducing a cleaning crew of good bacteria to your system, and you can expect to experience some digestive changes as that cleaning crew sets up shop. Hang in there for the first few days; the bacteria usually start to establish themselves quite quickly.

The Fab Five Fermented Foods

For the first week or so of incorporating fermented foods into their diet, I recommend people consume relatively small amounts of two of the following foods per day. (If a client is extremely sensitive, I recommend starting with just a teaspoon of one per day.) As their gut becomes stronger, I recommend increasing the amount, as listed below. Note that each food contains a different complement of bacteria, so it's good to eat a blend of the five, but if there's one you really don't like, don't panic. Some is better than none. And, as always, follow the Living in the Gray Guideline (see page 53).

- Kefir: ¼ cup to 1 cup
- Miso: 1 to 2 tablespoons
- Kimchi: 2 tablespoons to ½ cup
- Krauts, such as sauerkraut: 2 tablespoons to ½ cup
- Apple cider vinegar: 1 teaspoon to 2 tablespoons

Although I enjoy fermenting my own foods and love that more people are moving toward fermenting in their own kitchens, I understand that, for many people, there is a misunderstanding that fermented foods are spoiled. Often, clients send me photos of fermented foods—even foods they've purchased in the refrigerated section of the grocery store—because they want permission to eat foods that don't look the same as the foods they're used to eating. Relax. Fermented foods won't poison you. Do your best to avoid the fear factor and trust this natural, wild process.

Kefir

Kefir is fermented milk. Although it has a flavor similar to yogurt, it's different from yogurt primarily in that it hosts a wider range of bacteria. And while yogurt's bacteria is beneficial, it is typically transient bacteria, meaning that it passes through the body. Kefir's bacteria can colonize the gut, setting up camp there for the long term, which translates to more permanent benefits for the body. In addition, because bacteria break down the lactose in milk as they ferment it, most kefir is 99 percent lactose-free, making it a good option for many people with lactose intolerance.

Quick Ideas for Kefir

+ Drink it plain, before bedtime to help with sleep.
+ Make a post-workout smoothie by blending ½ cup kefir, 1 ripe banana, ½ cup full-fat coconut milk or whole milk, and ½ cup frozen or fresh blueberries, with enough additional whole milk to get the consistency you like.
+ Pour it over your granola or oatmeal.

I call kefir "nature's Prozac" because in addition to hosting beneficial bacteria, it's a natural source of the essential acid L-tryptophan. The body doesn't make L-tryptophan; we must ingest it from our food supply. Among other things, L-tryptophan stimulates the production of serotonin, a neurotransmitter that helps us feel better. (Serotonin increase is the end goal of most antidepressants.) L-tryptophan is also known to have a soothing effect; most of my clients notice an improvement in sleep patterns soon after they start drinking it (if they drink it at night before bed). It's not Ambien, but it does have a noticeable calming effect on the nervous system. Let's coin a new slogan: A half cup a day keeps the demons away.

You can make your own kefir from any type of milk, such as cow, goat, sheep, or even coconut milk, by adding kefir "grains." You can also buy prepared kefir in most natural grocery stores, either plain or flavored. While I would recommend kefir made with whole milk and less sugar, consuming it, regardless of what form it's in, is most important. I have had great success with clients who drink the sugary varieties. (Many people make the mistake of passing on healthy foods altogether if they aren't perfect. Try to move away from this black-and-white thinking.)

Miso

Miso is a rich, earthy fermented paste, most commonly used in Japanese cuisine as a flavoring agent. It's made from a blend of ingredients, usually including soybeans and sometimes grains but always with salt and a specific strain of "good" mold, that are fermented over the course of months or years. The fermentation process gives miso soup its namesake flavor (which I've heard well described as a mixture of salt, sea, and earth) and also creates a food packed with nutritional benefits.

Quick Ideas for Miso

- Stir a tablespoon into 2 cups bone broth and use it as a base for ramen or other noodle soups (don't forget to add the seaweed!).
- Shake together salad dressing made with equal parts miso, toasted sesame oil, rice vinegar, tahini, and olive oil.
- Spread it on a sandwich with tahini, avocado, sprouts, tomato, and arugula.
- Smear 1 tablespoon miso mixed with 1 tablespoon tamari on cooked salmon or chicken.
- Mix together 1 tablespoon each miso, apple butter, and peanut butter, and use as a spread for toast.
- Stir miso into mayonnaise to taste, and use it as a dip for sweet potato fries or artichokes.
- Find more recipes for miso on pages 225 and 234.

Miso was the first fermented food I incorporated into my diet on a regular basis, perhaps because it's easy to stir into almost anything and easy to find—that, and because I read about its ability to help prevent breast cancer, which took my mother's life. Although miso soup is traditionally made by stirring a lump of miso into dashi, a Japanese seaweed and fish broth, I rely often on miso soup made by stirring miso into previously frozen bone broth. It's a household staple when we return from traveling—because miso never goes bad, we always have it on hand. Even at typical grocery stores, it's common to find miso in multiple colors; try the one that appeals to you. (White miso is the most mellow.)

Remember, the bacteria in miso, as with kimchi and sauerkraut, die at too high a temperature. Add it to soups and stews only once they are cool enough to stick your finger into them comfortably.

Kimchi

Kimchi (also spelled kimchee), a staple of the Korean diet, was traditionally made of just cabbage. Over time, Western influence introduced spicy red peppers to the region; today, kimchi is made from a wide variety of vegetables and is often (though not always!) quite spicy. I first tried it in high school, eating at the home of my Korean boyfriend's family, who ate only traditional Korean foods, including kimchi and fermented beans. They served kimchi with each meal, using it as an accompaniment to everything. I happen to particularly like it with fried eggs for breakfast.

Traditional cabbage kimchi is nutrient-dense and packs a whopping dose of *lactobacillus plantarum*, a bacteria that serves as a cornerstone of good gut health. It also contains *Bacillus pumilus*, which is reportedly capable of dismantling the harmful chemical additive bisphenol A (BPA), a common environmental concern for families with young children. Buy kimchi in the refrigerated section of a natural grocery store.

Quick Ideas for Kimchi

- Use kimchi to top brown rice seasoned with butter, salt, and pepper.
- Serve baked potatoes with sour cream and kimchi.
- Top buttered toast with kimchi, then a fried egg and cheese. Broil just until the cheese melts.
- Substitute the liquid from a jar of kimchi for some of the vinegar in a salad dressing.
- Mix kimchi with peanut butter and enough warm water to create a tasty sauce for vegetables, rice, and meat.
- Add kimchi to a burger made with grass-fed beef and blue cheese.
- For another kimchi recipe, see page 220.

Krauts

Sauerkraut, like kimchi, is fermented cabbage containing immunity-boosting *lactobacillus plantarum*, a bacteria that helps the body digest lactose and reduce the growth of bad yeasts. Sauerkraut also contains the amino acid L-glutamine, which boosts gut and immune function and other essential processes in the body, especially during times of stress. (Some of my clients swear that their sauerkraut intake prevents them from getting sick in the winter.)

It's important to know, though, that the sauerkraut you find at a hot dog stand probably isn't the same sauerkraut as what you'll need to buy. Unrefrigerated sauerkraut doesn't contain any microbes, because that product has been pasteurized to within an inch of its life; I'm often surprised it has any flavor at all. I keep a Harsch crock—a German fermenting crock—on the back porch with sauerkraut going all year long. I love how forgiving it is; once you've followed a few simple steps putting the ingredients together, you can literally forget about it until you have sauerkraut waiting for you. That said, good sauerkraut teeming with beneficial bacteria is available in the grocery store. The label should read "raw" or "unpasteurized."

Today, many natural foods stores carry beet, carrot, and onion krauts, so venture off the traditional cabbage path if you're so inclined. The fermentation process is more important than the type of vegetable you're eating. The goal is to have 2 to 4 tablespoons per day on a regular basis, remembering not to get too rigid about doing anything every single day.

Quick Ideas for Sauerkraut

- Serve it traditionally, with sausages and potatoes.
- Add a small amount to the top of pancakes, with cinnamon and applesauce or apple butter.
- Dot pizza with spoonfuls of sauerkraut just before you eat it.
- Use it as a condiment for steak, roasted chicken, or pork chops.
- Layer well-drained sauerkraut into sandwiches (or stir it into tuna or chicken salad).
- Make Reuben-style sandwiches with grilled, sliced, grass-fed flank steak and pile them with kraut.

Apple Cider Vinegar

Apple cider vinegar is made by crushing apples, making apple juice, and then fermenting it. It's been used to cure a laundry list of ailments for decades. Because it's rich in B vitamins, vitamin C, and small amounts of important minerals, apple cider vinegar can soothe a sunburn, eradicate acne, and even protect against diabetes. (A study in *Annals of Nutrition and Metabolism* found that drinking a tablespoon of apple cider vinegar mixed with water before a meal reduced post-meal blood sugar in healthy people by about 20 percent and seemed to slow the release of sugar into the bloodstream.) Most notably, apple cider vinegar helps break down proteins in food, facilitating and improving digestion. And of course, the bacteria present in the vinegar help heal the gut.

To use apple cider vinegar, first make sure that the kind you buy is raw, unpasteurized vinegar. (It usually has a cloudy substance floating around near the bottom of the bottle, called the mother. You don't have to eat this.) Use it cold or add it to hot foods and beverages only once the temperature of the food is cool enough that you can stick your finger in it comfortably.

Quick Ideas for Apple Cider Vinegar

* Use apple cider vinegar for salad dressings, such as the Basic Apple Cider Vinaigrette on page 240.
* Mix 1 to 2 teaspoons of apple cider vinegar with a cup of hot water and a dollop of raw, local honey as a digestion-enhancing drink.
* Stir 1 to 2 tablespoons of apple cider vinegar into a pot of soup just before serving.
* Add a splash of apple cider vinegar to water, to brighten it.
* You'll find more recipes that include apple cider vinegar on pages 218, 222, 233, 235, 236, 237, 240 and 241.

Gut Goal #5: Practice Mindful Eating

I remember a construction worker with an acid reflux issue. He came in complaining that his belly ached after he ate, and he felt uncomfortable for hours after most meals. He wanted to change his diet in a way that allowed him to stop taking his acid reflux medication, in part because it was so expensive. He found that if he simply sat in his truck and ate lunch with music he liked, the reflux disappeared. Over the course of a few weeks, with a doctor's help, he weaned himself off his medication completely.

When we think about changing our diet, we think *what*, not *how*. It's much easier for people to incorporate new, sometimes crazy-sounding foods into their diet than it is to change the way they actually eat, but the latter is often more immediately rewarding. Eighty percent of my clients see me for weight loss, not debilitating digestive disorders. But for people who struggle with weight, changes in digestion are just as important as for those with irritable bowel syndrome, and slowing down at the table (or, more realistically, learning to sit down at a table first and then slowing down) is a huge step toward weight control. Eating under stress—something we are all familiar with in our too-busy lives—inhibits the production of the enzymes and hydrochloric acid that are necessary for proper digestion. If you're stressed, preoccupied, or rushing, if possible, try to avoid eating until you can sit down and give it your full attention. That sounds drastic, I know, but I guarantee you'll see and feel the results.

The stomach also has a limited capacity for digestion. Overeating decreases the effectiveness of its hydrochloric acid and digestive enzymes, causing discomfort and poor digestion. Often, the problem isn't that we naturally want to eat too much, but that we eat too quickly, so the brain doesn't have time to tell the stomach that it's full. If we eat mindfully, the brain can accurately monitor food intake and let us know when we've had enough.

Think of it this way: Food is our energy source. Assuming we are digesting well and eating the foods that are right for our body, we should eat so that we feel invigorated, not tired and sluggish. (Have you ever noticed how children tend to jump up from the lunch table, zinging with energy, because they've eaten just the right amount?) Overeating is, in effect, a way of self-medicating; it often sedates us and allows us to avoid the aspects of life that aren't as savory. Try eating until you're three-quarters full, leaving room in the stomach for the digestion required to turn food into energy.

It's also important to *enjoy* eating. This sounds obvious, right? But for many of my clients, most of whom swear that their chief problem is "loving food too much," it's rare that they remember the last time they've spent a full day eating all three meals away from the car, computer, television, or street. If you really love food, give it the attention and respect it deserves. Focus on it, and nothing else, while you enjoy it. When you go for the ice cream, put it in a bowl. Sit down. Savor every bite.

That said, we're human. Of course we all overeat sometimes—and sometimes, we have to eat on the go. Just be as aware as you can of how you eat (most of the time, of course).

Mindful Eating

Many of my clients—busy, determined people with successful careers and full lives—report eating so quickly that they often don't taste their food. Eating mindfully not only reduces stress (which effectively shuts down our digestion process), it also helps us develop the natural intuition required to balance what we need with what we eat, which I'll discuss in more detail in Chapter 8. Practice mindful eating by incorporating these simple digestion-improving tactics during your meals:

- Sit down to eat.
- Put down your fork between bites.
- Play slow music to set the tone.
- Try using chopsticks or eating with the opposite hand.
- Thoroughly chew each bite of food.
- Describe your foods' textures and flavors in your mind as you chew.
- Hold a secret competition with yourself to eat slower than someone else at the table.

A Gutsy Diet

It's ironic, I think, that my "untreatable" health problems—the gut pain that caused my doctors so much head-scratching (and caused me so much agony)—were what led me, in part, on a path toward nutrition as a career. And it's more ironic still that for so many people looking to lose weight and feel better, the very foods they focus on to become healthier are actually hurting them. They go around and around, trying medication after medication, diet after diet.

Ultimately, I think people come to Passionate Nutrition because they know, deep in their gut, that something has to change there. (We call it "gut instinct" for a reason; our guts have an intelligence that sometimes surpasses our brain's.) Sometimes people visit after a major event—a heart attack or news of a friend's cancer—but more often than not, it's a gut-wrenching, soul-crushing unhappiness that leads people to our doors. They come as a last resort. We recognize that for most, weight loss is the number one goal. And believe me, we see weight loss. But we always, always start with changes to the gut, in part because I believe that's the foundation of health, the source of weight loss, and where happiness is rooted.

So yes, it takes guts, so to speak, to focus on adding foods to your diet and trying new foods when you're looking for weight loss or have a debilitating health issue. Call it the "Gutsy Diet," if you want. But working my Five Goals for a Good Gut into your everyday life can dramatically change the way you feel and look. As always, when it comes to finding the perfect mix of the five for your own body, use your gut instinct. The best determinant of what's right for you is *you*.

....

THE PRESCRIPTION

- Eat gentle foods. Try it for one week and see how your body responds. Remember to listen to your body and not your brain. You will survive without salad for a week.
- Drink bone broth. If you have severe digestive issues, drink one to three cups per day if possible, but remember that anything is better than nothing. Aim for most of the time. For general purposes, use it when you are making soups, stews, or anything that calls for water.
- Introduce some of the Fab Five fermented foods. Aim to incorporate one or two fermented foods per day, most of the time.

Chapter 5

THE PROTEIN-SUGAR CONNECTION

com·pul·sive (kəm ′pəl siv) adj.
1. resulting from or relating to an irresistible urge,
especially one that is against one's conscious wishes.

Okay, so here's the thing: Late at night, when you're slumped against the kitchen wall with a pint of ice cream in one hand and a serving spoon in the other, you're probably thinking that you're the only person on the planet who doesn't have the willpower to just turn out the kitchen light and go to bed. You're not alone. Millions of people—including me—find themselves roaming the refrigerator not because they're defective, weak willed, tired, or lazy (all of which my clients report feeling). It's because they're *hungry*.

When we're hungry, we're not usually very nice to anyone, especially not ourselves. Catching ourselves eating "forbidden" foods can cause a cascade of mental self-flagellation. We beat ourselves up, using words and phrases meaner and more hurtful than anything we'd say to a sworn enemy.

You lazy, fat cow, why did you have to eat Cheryl's nasty cookies at the meeting? Can't you learn to say no? Or are you too goddamned stupid? And you had to have three. By the time we leave work, we've obliterated our self-worth by talking down to ourselves. While we're busy overthinking things on the way home from work, promising we'll never overeat again, planning the next diet, an alien takes over our body, forces the car to exit the highway, and suddenly we're buying a triple scoop of salted caramel ice cream. Sugar has taken control of the wheel, like it did yesterday and the day before that.

When a client comes to me reporting constant sugar cravings, I don't ban the offending foods, no matter how far they stray from the 100-Year Diet. Instead, I ask clients to add protein, and over the years, I've found that adding foods like chicken, beef, and eggs during the day cuts down on the wild-eyed, late-night refrigerator raids and sugar pit stops so many of us fear. It sounds crazy to treat a yearning for one thing with something so seemingly unrelated, I know. But that's just it: Eating protein helps prevent sugar cravings. If you get enough protein, you will not crave sugar in the same way.

Researchers can now explain why. A 2009 Bolivian study showed that spider monkeys base their diet on how much protein they get—that is, they eat and eat and eat until they get enough protein each day, no matter how much it means they eat altogether. Now attention has turned toward protein intake in humans. As my practice has confirmed over and over again, a 2011 Australian study also showed humans do the same thing. In that case, subjects put on a protein-limited diet ate more than their peers. Although it's clear that test subjects (and certainly spider monkeys) don't live in our lives, with our stresses, refrigerators, and ice cream (or in my case, chocolate) habits, they point to something important: We don't naturally eat until we're full. We eat until we've gotten exactly what our body needs, which includes protein. Because weight-loss efforts often focus on low-fat foods, and because many protein-rich foods are higher in fat, people on diets often don't get enough protein—and because the body isn't getting enough, the brain takes over and the diet fails. No wonder so many of us have been around the diet cycle so many times.

Eating protein during the day makes us feel full and sated, which helps prevent our bodies from flipping into desperation mode. In this chapter, I'll discuss the link between protein and sugar, and give you simple ideas for how to add protein to your diet in ways that cut down on cravings. (Eating protein has nutritional bonus points too: When we use protein as medicine to make us feel better, the "side effects" are undeniably enjoyable. Because protein makes up the building blocks for our physical body, increasing intake usually results in more energy and shinier, fuller hair. Put *that* on a pill bottle.)

What's Protein?

Growing up, I didn't know what protein was—that it existed in some foods but not in others, that it was something our bodies need, and (certainly not) that it balances blood sugar, regulates hormones, and maintains healthy muscles, skin, hair, and bones. Saying I lived off sugar as a teenager is not an exaggeration. Not surprisingly, throughout my youth, I was tired, emotional, and had huge sugar cravings. (When I ate cake, I sometimes ate just the frosting, because the cake itself wasn't sweet enough.) I never connected what I ate with how I felt. Looking back, it's clear I was simply not getting enough protein.

In the United States, we have a very confused idea of what protein means and how much we need. We hear from raw foodists that we can get enough protein from eating spinach. (I think that's technically possible, but considering that a cup of spinach has just .9 grams of protein, we'd have to resort to spending most of the day eating, like most primates do.) Also, we hear that Americans on the whole consume too much protein. I lived in the Midwest for a while, where I saw some serious protein intake, but the average American only gets about 15 percent of his or her dietary calories from protein, which is on the low side of the USDA and

World Health Organization's recommended dietary guidelines of between 10 and 35 percent.

Obviously, everyone has different protein needs, just like everyone has different food preferences; our bodies all function in unique ways. But we all *need* protein. From a scientific perspective, when we eat protein, the body breaks it down into smaller particles called amino acids. Our digestive tract is designed to absorb amino acids and pass them along to the bloodstream, which carries them to different parts of the body to help the nervous and immune systems; regulate hormones; maintain muscles, bones, skin, and hair; and balance blood sugar.

From a very nonscientific perspective, the body is a giant glob of protein and water. We all know we can't survive long without water. Likewise, when we don't get enough protein, we feel stressed, anxious, tired, and unable to concentrate. In a way, our body starves.

Over the course of my practice, I've noticed that adding protein throughout the day is the key to making it through. (Not surprisingly, studies are now showing that the protein requirement numbers we've depended on for so long are vastly underestimated.) Many dieters skip or skimp on breakfast, which sets them up for sugar cravings later in the day because right off the bat, their bodies haven't been nourished enough to make it until noon. When they eat a huge salad for lunch, minus the meat, they effectively point their bodies toward a predictable afternoon crash. Even after a dinner containing some sort of meat or fish, those who limit protein during the day inevitably face a problem in their pajamas: Their body hasn't gotten enough protein. They need something quick and delicious, because their body feels deprived and hungry for instant gratification. Cue the cupcakes.

Adding protein to a client's diet is the rare time I feel like a rock star. Usually, I take a slow, steady approach and coach clients on practicing patience. Protein is different. Because people usually notice a difference in their eating habits within three days, and because adding protein can be extremely enjoyable, clients come back raving about how much of a difference protein has made in their lives. Consuming a protein-rich breakfast, protein at lunch, and a protein-heavy snack around three p.m. transforms a person's energy levels and creates a natural control for sugar cravings.

How Much Protein Is Enough?

Protein gives us power, both literally, in the sense that it fuels our cells, and figuratively, in that consuming it allows us to regain control over what we eat. Unfortunately, some people are confused about or afraid of eating protein, either because they don't know which foods contain it or they think protein-rich foods contain too much fat or that they can't afford it. Perhaps I should offer a clarification: I'm not asking you to order a rib eye for lunch every day. I'm not telling you to roast a whole chicken for dinner every night. Meeting our protein requirements doesn't mean switching our overeating from sugary foods to meat; it means incorporating protein into our lives in a balanced way, on a regular basis, and all day long—in order of importance, in the morning, at noon, and in the afternoon.

I hope you know by now that I'm not a stickler for numbers. I advocate listening to body wisdom over counting calories or grams every time. But if you're concerned about sugar cravings, try calculating how much protein you take in over the course of three days, because you may be surprised by just how much protein you require.

An average 160-pound person, for example, needs about 80 grams of protein per day, on the low side. To put this in perspective, that means in one day, you'd need to eat 1 egg (7 grams), 1 cup of beans (14 grams), 1 cup of milk (8 grams), ¼ cup of nuts (8 grams), and 6 ounces of meat, poultry, or fish (42 grams, from a piece about the size of two decks of cards). That puts you on the lower end of the range of protein you might need, and just barely. An extremely active person needs twice that much, and many of us fall somewhere in between. If you already eat protein, this probably sounds doable, but for many of the dieters who enter Passionate Nutrition, adding up the amount of protein they currently get in their diet often reveals that they're eating protein levels akin to someone in a developing country.

It's no wonder they feel starved all the time. They don't need willpower; they need food.

Go-To Energy Boosters

Choosing easy breakfast and lunch options with protein in them and packing high-protein midafternoon snacks is crucial to balancing energy throughout the day without spending too much time in the kitchen. I know you may be surprised by the fat content of some of the ideas below. I'll discuss fat in more detail in the next few chapters, but for now, trust that it will help you achieve your goals.

Breakfast:
- Egg frittata
- Egg, sausage, and cheese English muffin sandwiches
- Deli meat roll-ups with avocado
- Poached eggs with toast
- Cottage cheese and berries
- Sausage links and sauerkraut
- Miso soup with eggs or fish (traditional Japanese breakfast)
- Oatmeal with 1 whisked raw egg per serving (stir it into the raw oatmeal and cook the oatmeal as usual)

Lunch:
- Turkey wraps, made by spreading cream cheese on turkey slices, then wrapping avocado, tomato, and sprouts up inside
- Sausage with sauerkraut and pickles
- Lettuce wraps with meat or fish and vegetables, dipped in salad dressing or peanut sauce
- Collard greens wrapped around chicken, tuna, or egg salad
- Chicken, tuna, or salmon salad made with sour cream, apples, and walnuts
- Leftover rotisserie chicken and sautéed vegetables
- Tuna and white bean salad

Snacks:
- Hard-boiled or deviled eggs
- Nuts or seeds
- Cheese slices
- Tinned sardines on crackers
- Beef jerky
- Tinned oysters, mussels, or clams
- Turkey, roast beef, or chicken roll-ups with cream cheese, avocado, and sprouts

---

Food is meant to be enjoyed, not measured, but just this once, I'd like you to get out your trusty math skills. Don't open an Excel spreadsheet; for this exercise, you need a pen and a napkin or a sticky note, if that. For three days, keep track, even with rough estimates, of how much protein (in grams) you're getting every day.

There are entire books devoted to determining how much protein you need. I agree with those that say we need .8 grams to 1 gram of protein per kilogram of body weight, depending on your body and activity level, but I simplify the calculation. To determine how many grams of protein you need each day, divide your body weight in pounds by half. If you weigh 180 pounds, you need 90 grams of protein per day. If you weigh 150 pounds, you need 75 grams. As you begin your three-day math project, gauge whether you're over or under your estimated protein requirement. Now, forget the math. Throw the napkin or the sticky note far, far away.

This is an oversimplified approach to how much protein each body requires to function, but it offers a good, simple guideline. We've all read how unhealthy Americans are and how much we overconsume protein. As a result, our reaction is to cut back on it when we try to lose weight. We may shed the pounds initially, but we also lose energy, muscle mass, hair, and immune function, and eventually begin craving sugar because we need fast energy, which typically brings back the weight we're trying so hard to lose. If this all sounds awfully familiar to you, take a close look at your protein intake. For many people, this sounds crazy, I understand. Many long-term dieters have trained themselves to avoid things like meat and eggs. Try it for three days. (Remember, for most people, increasing protein brings dramatic changes in energy and sugar cravings quickly, usually within just a few days. This is rare in the world of nutritional changes, so revel in it.)

Not All Protein Is Created Equal

Throughout my twenties, when almost every medical provider I saw admonished me for not eating enough protein, I knew they were right. But I was a strict vegetarian; I ate legumes, tofu, nuts, and the occasional egg. Even considering ingesting animal meat threw me into a total emotional panic. I'd worked at The Little Nell in Aspen, one of the best restaurants in the country, and stuck to my vegetarian diet despite it being world renowned for its meat preparations. For me, vegetarianism was a moral issue; after watching livestock being butchered as a child in Missouri, I firmly turned against eating meat at thirteen. I just couldn't bring myself to eat it. But looking back, recognizing the lethargy and depression I now know I suffered from a very early age, I recognize my kind-hearted kid compassion prevented me from thriving when I had access to food.

Today, I tell most of my clients to get enough protein, with an emphasis on animal protein. (As an aside, I also tell my vegetarian friends to introduce their children to meat and let them make their own decisions about food values later in life.) For adults, teens, and children alike, I have found that animal proteins do a better job of curbing carbohydrate and sugar cravings, increasing energy, helping with anxiety and depression, and aiding in weight loss. In fact, when vegetarians come in with sugar cravings, increasing their protein intake usually helps with sugar cravings but doesn't always take them away as effectively as it might if they ate animal meat.

Animal proteins work best because they are more bioavailable than plant proteins, meaning the body is able to absorb and use them efficiently. Like us, plants are engineered to survive by protecting themselves, but, frankly, plants are a lot more resilient than we are. Seeds want to grow up as plants instead of being pulverized inside our bodies. As a result, plant cell membranes are tougher, which is why we have a harder time extracting nutrients from them. Plants also contain phytates, which prevent mineral absorption in humans. (Interestingly, cows can digest phytates, which is why they can subsist on a vegetarian diet. Well, that, and that they eat, digest, and redigest all day long. Score one for the quadruple stomach.)

Also, although many vegetarians do a good job eating vegetables, they usually consume far too many carbohydrates overall, which results in nutritional imbalance and, often, low energy, sugar cravings, and weight gain. If a person eating a vegetarian diet for weight management isn't getting enough protein, it's likely that he or she has low muscle mass. Since muscle is more metabolically active (i.e. burns more calories) than other parts of the body, adding meat to the diet usually results in weight loss. I'm certainly not saying beans and lentils are bad for you, but animal protein offers a much more reliable path toward immediate changes in energy and body function. After years of practice (and thirteen years of living as a vegetarian), I simply can't say the same for plant-based protein.

Naturally, when a woman comes into my office with "VEGAN" tattooed across her midsection, I'm not going to attack her core belief system. In her case, I'll work with her to maximize the nutritional benefits she can find with just plant proteins and help her learn the discipline required to balance a vegan diet. (Although it's possible, it's a pretty stressful way to live.) But when a client says he's a vegetarian "for health reasons," we do often review the health benefits of vegetarianism and compare them to the benefits of eating meat. And in my experience, eating a broader range of proteins almost always wins.

If you're a vegetarian with glowing skin, abundant energy, stable moods, and no sugar cravings, I will most likely not see you in my office. For now, vegetarianism works for you, which is great. Eat on. But if you are a vegan or vegetarian whose health is suffering, and eating the right amount of protein isn't helping with fatigue and sugar cravings, be open to the possibility that your body likely *needs* meat. You might be surprised, like I was, by how much adding meat to your diet can change your life.

For me, the transition from vegetarian to carnivore wasn't easy. And I'll let you in on a little secret: I still don't love meat all that much. First, there's the killing thing, which, even though I now eat meat, I haven't totally gotten over. But I choose beef that's been grass-fed using sustainable ranching practices and chicken that's been pastured. I know the animals I buy have led happy, natural lives, which helps me a lot. Because I've found farmers I trust to treat (and kill) animals humanely, the moral issue is no longer as strong for me. (As an aside, buying well-raised animals also allows me to vote with my fork. When I eat pastured meat, I am supporting the farmers who go against the grain, so to speak.)

The other thing I've learned is that I really do enjoy meat when I mix it into things—beef in bean tacos or pasta sauces, for example, or soup with chopped chicken in it. Even adding small portions to a meal I used to make without meat can make a huge difference. Often, we see that vegetarian clients

Beef: A Bad Rap

Although the press has vilified red meat over the last few decades, it's important to recognize that beef quality varies wildly based on what the animals eat and how they're raised. While feedlot beef can indeed be quite fatty, inflammatory, and hard to digest, grass-fed beef has a radically different nutritional profile, including much higher levels of essential fatty acids, which are, as the name implies, essential for life's myriad functions. If you're terrified of eating beef simply because you've been conditioned for decades to believe that it's bad for you, consider grass-fed beef a different food. (Given its nutritional profile, it certainly acts like a different food inside our bodies.) It's more expensive, but you don't need to eat a lot, and there are less expensive cuts.

Similarly, many people avoid beef because it's known to contain cholesterol, which has been linked in the past to heart disease. What the $31-billion-a-year cholesterol drug industry doesn't explain when they warn doctors of the dangers of high cholesterol levels is that inflammation, high glycemic levels, and belly fat also play huge roles—the leading roles—in determining heart health. Add to that the important part cholesterol plays in preventing metabolic syndrome (the term the Centers for Disease Control and Prevention uses for the insulin-resistant condition considered a precursor to heart disease and type 2 diabetes) and regulating sex hormones (which I'll address in detail in Chapter 10), and a steak suddenly sounds like a good idea. Take what you hear about lowering cholesterol with a grain of salt. Cholesterol is not the big issue. If you're limiting beef because you're concerned about heart disease, remember that what you're eating—perhaps a diet high in refined carbohydrates and low in natural fats—could be more dangerous than what you aren't.

are more able to eat meat if it is blended into their regular food because they feel so much better (but don't actually have to use a steak knife).

For carnivores, the type of meat we eat affects us as well. Although it's not common practice in the United States, traditional forms of medicine always consider the energetics of food; energy from cow meat affects us differently than energy from chicken meat, for example. When I walk into a room full of people I've never met, I can often tell within the first few minutes of talking to them what types of meat proteins people eat by the way they act. Nervous, flighty women with lots of sparkly jewelry typically eat a ton of chicken. Slow-talking, methodical folks are beef eaters. Determined, self-preserving types or natural dissidents are often big fish eaters; they swim upstream. Conversely, when clients are looking to add certain components to their life, I recommend they consider the meats they're eating. If they need more calm, I recommend beef. If they need more energy, I recommend chicken. If they need perseverance, I recommend cold-water fish. It may sound hokey, but I personally tend to be a little floaty and sometimes frantic, so I use what I call "cow energy" to keep calm and grounded. (Chicken is the last thing I need.) Try it. You might be surprised.

It's Not You, It's Sugar

So you've started eating more protein. Congrats! Chances are good that you've kicked the afternoon doldrums by eating more at breakfast and lunch and adding protein-centric afternoon snacks. (Notice a trend here: I'm still asking you to add foods, not take them away.) Chances are it also felt strange, because changing eating habits isn't as easy as it sounds. (If it were, you'd be reading something else.) No matter what choices you make about eating protein, though, there's still a chance that stubborn sugar cravings will persist. Hear this: It's not your fault. Studies show that sugar is eight times as addictive as cocaine. Likely without realizing it, you're consuming a food that is, in effect, a drug. That sugar can be as addicting as an illegal substance sounds like an overstatement, but when clients sit down in my office, emotionally crippled because they have run out of strategies for controlling their constant cravings for sweet things, the symptoms I see are often not of people who have no willpower, but of people who are, in a word, hooked.

A pair of 2013 Connecticut College studies showed that the part of rats' brains that respond to pleasure—the same portion often studied in connection to addiction—responded more strongly to an Oreo prize at the end of a maze than they did to an injection of morphine or cocaine. The research doesn't prove that Oreos are addictive, but it certainly suggests certain sugary foods launch strong positive physiological reactions. When a different study gave already cocaine-addicted rats the choice between more cocaine and sugar water, forty out of forty-three rats chose the sugar water.

Sugar rules us. When we ingest sugar, our insulin and dopamine levels spike, and the body starts a series of inflammatory reactions, often resulting in foggy thinking and mood swings. In an understandable effort to combat the inevitable fatigue that follows, we eat more sugar, often relying on processed foods (since it's not really mealtime), which often contain added sugar. Add to the suite of sweets that tempt us daily, the kinds of chemicals the modern food industry adds to foods to make them actually addictive— none of which contain the protein the body needs to feel full—and we're basically goners. As mortal humans, we never stood a chance against a food industry channeling billions of dollars into finding the bliss point (the point at which pleasure and enjoyment are at their absolute peak) of packaged foods and drinks.

Some people question whether sugar as a food additive could gain FDA approval if it needed to today. From a political standpoint, I'm sure it would, because so much of our politicians' corporate financial support comes from companies that rely on sugar for profit. Big Sugar has become the new Big Tobacco. As reported in the documentary *Fed Up*, of the 600,000 food items available for sale in America, 80 percent contain added sugar, yet on a (government-designed) nutrition label, there is no percent daily value (% DV) number entered for sugar. In other words, the government will tell us we're getting, say, 30 grams of sugar in one serving of cola, but fails to tell us that one cola alone is way more than most health sources recommend. (The USDA makes no firm sugar recommendation.) The movie also pointed out that sugar can be so dangerous that the World Health Organization, which suggests limiting sugar to 25 grams per day, has issued a call for a 50 percent reduction in sugar consumption worldwide. So far, the United States is ignoring it.

When I work with clients on sugar cravings, I always start by balancing the body's physiology first, because that alone can eliminate sugar cravings. (Many of my clients are referred from psychologists, who want me to address their patients' nutritional needs first to help define where their emotional issues really lie.) But I understand that sugar has an emotionally addicting side too. When someone tells us we can't have something, it's natural to want it. Clients tell me over and over that sugar seems as addictive as smoking. That they'd dash across a highway at rush hour for a quick dessert. That they often put sweet things above work and family, because they *need* them. Perhaps you've felt this way. The problem isn't you. The problem is sugar.

More pragmatically, sugar is usually quite convenient in our culture. When we need a break from work or chores, it's quick and easy to munch on something sugary—chocolate, sweet "fruit" snacks, baked goods, and candy are easy to eat on the go or at our desks. No wonder we become addicted in the first place. It's everywhere.

Another important step toward moving away from binging on sugary foods is recognizing that sugar (along with salt and fat) is a flavor we are engineered to love. Sugar signals safety. We are programmed to know that sweet flavors indicate a food is not poisonous, which is something our ancestors had to worry about. We're human. Let yourself be human too. It's okay to *like* and *ingest* sugar; we just want to move away from addiction. I'll talk more about the emotional side of sugar and how to create a healthier relationship with your "forbidden" foods in Chapter 8.

Bacteria Beat Sugar

If you've adjusted your protein intake and started to understand why we pine for sugar, but you still struggle, there are other strategies that work to decrease cravings. And—you guessed it—those cravings have more to do with what's going on down in our gut than what's up in our head.

When we crave sugar, it's often not really *us* craving the sugar, but rather a kind of bacteria I haven't talked about yet. We all have probiotics in our body—the "good" bacteria I talked about in Chapter 4—that reduce intestinal inflammation, digest lactose and protein, manufacture vitamins, make short-chain fatty acids, and help break down and eliminate toxins. We all also have "bad" bacteria in our body. (Saying they're "good" and "bad" is overly simplified, but it illustrates the point that we don't use all bacteria in the same way.) Like us, the bad bacteria are all about survival. They live off sugar, which we happily provide, in the form of both natural and added sugars. The more we feed them, the more they grow and multiply, and the more they signal to our bodies that they need more food, which in their case means more sugar. By feeding the gut's good bacteria and encouraging them to take over the bad bacteria, we can effectively control the amount of sugar our body tells our brain it needs.

Remember that while we may often think we're in charge of our bodies and our cravings, biology—and specifically, bacteria—has much more power than we do. I realized this most profoundly about a decade ago when, in an effort to offer a friend emotional support, and as an experiment, I joined her on a two-week sugar cleanse. We avoided sugar—no added sugars, but also none of the sugars found naturally in foods such as carrots and beets. By that time, my physiology had changed, and I no longer craved sugar like I used to, but still, I noticed a huge difference in my body. As the bad bacteria starved from lack of the natural sugars I normally consume every day, I developed debilitating sugar cravings, followed by headaches, mood swings, and fatigue—all indicating that while we think we may have the willpower to control what we take in, on many levels, we have nothing to do with it.

Starving the bad bacteria made me feel horrible and showed me how little power I had over them as they fought for survival. I blamed myself. Even though I knew better, I chastised myself for lacking willpower. But wanting sugar is rarely about willpower; it's about physiology. Bacteria run the show, so taking care of ourselves requires taking care of them. (A side note: In general, I don't recommend cleanses, because they're often too restrictive and cause a yo-yo effect.)

Besides controlling bad bacteria, consuming good bacteria can also make us happier. Ninety-five percent of the body's serotonin, for example, which helps regulate mood, is created by good bacteria in the gut.

Maintaining good gut health, as I discussed in Chapter 4, can boost serotonin, and lift our mood. I call Kefir "nature's Prozac" because it's especially high in tryptophan (as discussed on page 81). Adding things like the Fab Five fermented foods (outlined on page 80) can have a huge physiological impact on our need for sugary foods.

The Protein-Sugar Connection

When clients come in, they sometimes back up what they see as a character flaw—loving and craving sugar—by blaming their families for their eating habits. "My mother worked, so we ate a lot of packaged food," they'll say with a helpless, hopeless shrug. "I come from a typical American family." The subtext is that while their mothers and fathers may have set excellent examples as parents, they set poor dietary examples, and the clients are thus doomed to loving sweets and battling them on a daily basis, for the rest of their life. You might have a hard time seeing that sugar addiction is something that can change. You might not see yet that loving sugar isn't your (or your family's) fault. But believe me, it can change. And it isn't your fault.

I come from donuts, people. I come from donuts and cake and packaged macaroons, and from tubs of pre-made frosting and stolen Snickers bars.

I was a cake-and-french fries vegetarian for thirteen years. And while I admit that I haven't struggled with weight the way many of my clients have, I have certainly grappled with being desperately, painfully hungry and addicted. I know what it feels like to *need* sugar. I spent years stealing sugary foods. I understand now, of course, that there was a powerful physiological need behind my cravings. I've made the protein-sugar connection.

The change you feel when you start eating enough protein may surprise you. For me, it was night and day. You'll likely feel increased energy, reliable satiety, and decreased sugar cravings—but perhaps most significantly, a huge drop in the inevitable stress involved in being constantly angry with yourself for eating too many sweets. People—but women especially—spend a lot of energy blaming themselves, for everything from their plants dying to their kid's bad attitudes to their own eating habits. Shame rules our lives. Understanding your physiology with regard to sugar, and changing it by increasing protein, will hopefully help you learn that even though you may have spent decades hating yourself for eating sugar, it's not your fault.

I hear you: You're nervous. You're eating protein, sure, and it makes you feel better. But you're eating more fat now. You're thinking, *will I gain weight?* For now, trust how much better you feel. We will discuss the important role of fats in Chapter 8.

....

THE PRESCRIPTION

- Feel better about yourself knowing that sugar cravings are a biological response to physiological needs, not a lack of willpower.
- Adjust your diet to include enough protein throughout the day, preferably animal protein, especially early in the day. Focus on breakfast, lunch, and daytime snacks. Dinner and evening snacks are less important.
- Get enough beneficial bacteria (probiotics), such as kefir, to help keep your gut's sugar-loving bacteria in check.

Chapter 6

WEIGHT LOSS *and*
the METABOLISM MIRACLE

You can have it all. Just not all at once.

—Oprah Winfrey

When Jeanine came to Passionate Nutrition for the first time, she sort of spilled into my office. She carried with her, in overstuffed bags, binders, and envelopes, the evidence of a lifetime of dieting. She opened all her various toting devices and slowly stacked folders and notebooks on my desk, pausing so I could see how she'd carefully labeled each one. There was evidence of Atkins, South Beach, macrobiotic, raw, Weight Watchers, Paleo, fat-free, HCG, and Zone diets. As she reached the bottom of a canvas tote, I saw traces of old-school grapefruit and cabbage soup diets. Finally, she sat. "I've tried everything," she swore, dropping her curly blonde head into her hands. She said she was only forty and couldn't imagine dealing with such an overwhelming sense of failure much longer. "I've succeeded at *nothing*. Food is my enemy." The tears flowed.

That there's a connection between dieting and personal failure is a common misconception among people trying to lose weight. But inevitably, it's there. Eighty percent of my clients come in for weight loss. They've tried diet after diet, usually losing weight initially, only to gain it all (or more) back, always with a sense of crushing defeat. No wonder we feel like we've failed. When we employ restrictive dieting techniques, we set our bodies up for feelings of deprivation and starvation. It's Don Quixote attacking the windmill; we create goals we are often physically incapable of achieving. No one should live on 500 calories a day, ever. Even a third of people who undergo bariatric surgery, which I don't recommend, regain the weight they lose within two years of the procedure.

At the end of our session, I told Jeanine to have a bonfire with everything she had brought into my office—not because her past struggles weren't worth recognizing, but because I wanted her to feel liberated from what she considered her past failures, free of numbers and the shame she reported feeling every time she reached the end of a day a few bites (or a full-on binge) over her goals. I wanted her to start over feeling hope for a new future, not just physically, but mentally, knowing that she wouldn't have to repeat the diet cycles of the past. I wanted her to have a chance at loving herself instead of hating herself.

I recognize why my clients are attracted to fad diets. It's normal to be impatient, to want weight loss *now*, to wake up in the morning with dread when we remember the previous night's excesses or the last diet's failure, and to dream that eating just meat or no meat or just carbs or no carbs will make us thin, energetic, and sane for the first time in decades. We want a magic pill because we feel sick. Sick, and often utterly heartbroken.

The thing about "magic," in the form of quick weight-loss plans, is that it's crazy making. Spending hours each day tracking calories, looking at food in terms of numbers instead of pleasure and enjoyment, is not a human (or humane) way to live. It turns you into a robot. It compounds the profound sadness many people struggling with weight feel. Diets emphasize failure every single day, so they crush us emotionally. And worse, from a physiological perspective, they don't work.

In the *New York Times*, health writer Tara Parker-Pope labeled the awful diet cycle so many have endured "the Fat Trap," which is accurate, both emotionally and physiologically. "Anyone who has ever dieted knows that lost pounds often return, and most of us assume the reason is a lack of discipline or a failure of willpower," she says. She goes on to explain that weight loss, especially quick weight loss, causes the body to "defend" the old, higher weight by craving more calories than the lower body weight needs. In other words, a body that's used to starving learns to hoard calories, even when it doesn't need them. Fast off, fast on, as Mr. Miyagi (from *The Karate Kid*) might have said. Dieting is a trap in the most literal sense of the word; we fall in and can't climb out.

If weight-loss dreams came true so quickly and easily, and in one attempt, as so many diets predict, the diet industry wouldn't be the $60 billion-a-year machine it is today. We wouldn't be a nation of lemmings chasing after one random person each year who touts the diet that happened to work really fast for them. I approach weight loss with an eye to the long term. Of course you want to look great in a swimsuit in two months; that's a normal thing to want. But ultimately, I want to help you lose weight in a way that's sustainable for the rest of your life, because there's no reason to go back to the diet cycle. First, I address your underlying physiological issues, adding foods that boost metabolism. Over time, your changing metabolism and increased general satiety will likely cause weight loss.

I will not ask you to count calories. I will not ask you to achieve unrealistic goals. It's a totally different approach, and it works without sucking the enjoyment out of life. Warning: This approach—or perhaps I should just say "food," because that's what we're really talking about using here, as medicine to help you change your weight—has side effects. You'll probably notice improved energy, happier moods, and better skin and hair. I might let you deal with those on your own.

While I'll wait until the next chapter to discuss our nation's absurdly distorted perception of health, I know that most of us want to get closer to our own body's ideal weight, whatever that may mean. (From my clients' perspectives, it usually means losing weight.) Here's the bombshell: The diets you've tried haven't worked because they focus on short-term goals and avoid food. We all need to eat, and we probably need to eat a lot more than you think. Contrary to conventional wisdom, cutting calories often leads to weight *gain*.

Seven Steps to Weight Loss

In the pages that follow, you'll learn why Passionate Nutrition's seven-step weight-loss plan (which, by the way, I don't usually present to our clients as such a formulaic prescription) will make you look and feel healthier, and help you find and sustain the weight that's right for your body.

1. Clean Up Your Diet

When you're choosing foods, the simple act of eating clean, by avoiding chemicals and steroids, can help you lose weight. Let's start with chemicals: Artificial sweeteners, which we often consume in an effort to lose weight, can actually cause weight gain. Research shows that artificially sweetened beverages, for example, are linked to greater body mass index (BMI), as well as an increased risk of metabolic syndrome and type 2 diabetes. While that diet soda may lack calories, it still signals an impending arrival of nutrients to your gut. The body anticipates feeling some sort of satiety. When no nutrients show up, your gut tells you to eat again, and you often end up eating more than you originally intended. So over time, drinking artificially sweetened beverages can weaken the cascade of physiological events that indicate satiety. Those daily Diet Cokes prevent your body from being able to tell that it's full.

While some doctors prescribe anti-obesity drugs (which have nasty side effects), very few recommend decreasing chemical consumption. I go directly to the source, promoting foods that aid metabolism and offer satiety rather than adding pills, which are effectively swallowable Band-Aids. (We all know that Band-Aids eventually fall off.) Steering away from overly processed, packaged foods and toward the 100-Year Diet described in Chapter 3 allows the body to burn stored fat more efficiently.

Avoiding steroids can also decrease weight. It's generally accepted that, like the steroids some athletes abuse, prescription steroids—the types used to treat many inflammatory and autoimmune diseases, such as various forms of arthritis—cause weight gain. Less well known is that it takes only a tiny amount of added steroids to alter hormone balance and those tiny amounts exist in many of the foods we eat. In the 1950s, the FDA began approving steroid hormone additives for livestock to help them gain weight by producing fat cells. While some hormones are now fed to conventional cattle on a regular basis, others are only used during discrete growth periods for beef, poultry, and pork. The hormones work; they make livestock bigger, and they make cows produce more milk. But when those steroids are passed on to us, in the meat or dairy we eat, our hormones change. Every meal counts, because even one meal containing hormone-tainted foods can encourage our bodies to hold on to fat. The more you focus on choosing good, grass-fed beef over conventional beef and organic, hormone-free dairy over conventional dairy, the fewer hormones you will consume secondhand.

A whole foods diet—one that avoids additives of all sorts and emphasizes eating foods in their natural state over processed foods—can also increase metabolism, and thus decrease weight, on its own, simply because eating whole foods means consuming foods high in fat-burning and metabolism-boosting nutrients. Chromium, for example, plays a critical role in controlling blood sugar, which in turn helps us metabolize food properly and efficiently. It's found in vegetables such as broccoli, green beans, and tomatoes, in whole grains such as oats and barley, and in black pepper and thyme—none of which are likely to be found in their natural state in a box of processed protein bars.

Similarly, magnesium helps regulate nutrient absorption. Low magnesium levels—common in diabetics—are linked to systemic inflammation and poor absorption of fat. Increasing magnesium intake allows the body to store and use fat properly, which often results in weight loss. Good dietary sources of magnesium include pumpkin seeds, cashews, sesame seeds, spinach, black beans, and quinoa. Likewise, B vitamins help convert food into the energy we need to feel fueled all day, and essential fatty acids increase metabolism. If your goal is weight loss, eat foods that are natural and nutrient dense. Those weight loss bars and drinks? In the trash. Hundred-calorie snack packs? Out the window. Eat food.

2. Add Bacteria to Your Diet

Remember, as I discussed in Chapter 4, that only about one in ten of the cells in the average human body is actually human. The rest are microbial, the vast majority of which are in the gut. Not surprisingly, their happy function there, hidden in that tennis court's worth of intestinal lining deep inside us, plays a crucial role in our weight. Bacteria help us coax calories out of the food we eat, which means that their very balance (in number and type) controls how many calories we get out of a given meal. The more we get out of each bite, the less we feel we need more food. Jeff Gordon, the scientist who showed how swapping the gut bacteria of normal weight and overweight mice resulted in the thin mice gaining weight and the obese mice losing weight (see page 78), reminds us that this means we don't all necessarily get the same calories out of a bowl of Cheerios or yogurt. Some of us simply glean more calories from foods not because of our own genes or habits, but because of how the *bacteria's* genes function. In other words, what scientists have coined the "metagenome"—the combination of our own genome plus that of all the microbes in our bodies—may have more of an effect on our weight than the amount of food we eat and our genes do. Bacteria help control weight. Use them to your advantage.

3. *Eat Adequate Protein*

In Chapter 5, I explained how eating enough protein can decrease sugar cravings. (You'll find a simple way to calculate about how much protein you need each day on page 95.) Protein also gives us the fuel we need to make it through the day. Eat it, and when you can, focus on animal proteins.

4. *Eat Adequate Fat*

The conventional wisdom of the last half century or so has held that if you eat fat, you get fat. That conventional wisdom is wrong. As Dr. Walter Willett of the Harvard School of Public Health has said, "Fat is not the problem."

Interestingly, fat wasn't considered a dietary concern before World War II. In the 1950s, a researcher named Ancel Keys authored a study of people in seven countries that concluded that fat (and specifically, cholesterol and saturated fat) were responsible for an uptick in cardiovascular disease in the early part of the century. His research, now questioned, led to a cascade of similar studies, most of which propelled the myth that saturated fats, found in animal fats, are bad for us. This so-called lipid hypothesis, which took root in the second part of the twentieth century, led to the popular belief that fat (in the form of blood cholesterol) leads to heart disease. Curiously, however, as US consumers switched to processed foods such as margarine and corn oil and moved away from using animal fats for cooking, heart disease skyrocketed and our waistlines expanded.

It's not an accident. Nutrition expert Gary Taubes explains in *Why We Get Fat* that metabolic syndrome—thought to be a precursor to heart disease and type 2 diabetes—is more likely a result of high insulin levels, which are in turn a result of eating too-high levels of carbohydrates. In other words, the processed and sugary foods we thought for decades were the key to health, such as sugar-filled fat-free yogurts, refined pasta, and low-fat crackers, are now thought to contribute to cardiovascular disease and weight gain.

Eating fat is also crucial for bone health, immunity, and satiety. When we restrict fat intake, the stomach effectively signals to the brain that we aren't getting what we need for optimum health, so our hunger continues, even if we're eating lots of low-fat foods. We never feel sated. As a result, we overeat, which often leads to discomfort and shame, and, of course, the inevitable blood sugar crash. Because we don't feel full, it makes sense that we give in to our cravings. Low-fat diets don't work because they take away something our body naturally both needs and craves. I can't count the number of times clients who've subsisted for years on food point systems lose weight when they start eating more, specifically eating more fat. (They typically get really mad once they realize how much time, energy, and money they've spent adding so much stress to their lives counting points.) Although there's no magic number when it comes to fat intake, it's important to consume some fat with every meal and snack we eat. (In my life, this translates to a lot of butter and cream, because I enjoy them, and I notice that these foods in particular make me feel full.)

I can hear you. "Listen to this! A nutritionist is saying that I can lose weight by eating more *butter*!" We've been so conditioned to avoid fat that being encouraged to eat it seems preposterous, but it's true: an increase in healthy fats (such as those rich in omega-3s, found in oily fish, pastured meats and dairy, nuts, and seeds) can lead to weight loss. I'll say it again, because if you've "been there, done that" with diets like so many of my clients have, it's hard to believe: an increase in fat consumption can lead to weight loss. (Note that I'm asking you to include fat in your diet, not subsist on it and nothing else.) But it's more important to recognize that, while fat plays a crucial role in the function of our immune and hormonal systems, we also lose weight by adding fat because when we eat fat, we avoid eating other things—namely, the loads of refined carbohydrates and processed foods we gravitate toward when we're not sated.

Again, it's easy to point a finger at the French. They eat croissants for breakfast and pâté at lunch. Dinner usually means what Americans might consider a holiday meal, often with multiple courses, followed by dessert and cheese. Yet their incidence of heart disease is far below ours, and they are much less likely to be overweight.

On the flip side, consider a 1930 "station bulletin," from Oregon State Agricultural College's Agricultural Experiment Station, entitled "Fattening Pigs for Market." It counsels farmers that a feed regimen combining skim milk, which provides protein but not fat, and grain, which is typically fat-free or extremely low in fat, is the best way to fatten a pig (because they're never sated, so they keep eating). So basically, the low-fat diet we've been conditioned to embrace over the last half century is the same one farmers used to fatten pigs almost a century ago. Coincidence? I think not. Redefine what you think it might mean to eat like a pig.

From my perspective, the general health of the French is not at all surprising, and neither is the size of the conventional pork industry's pigs. Eating enough fat ensures fewer cravings, less overeating, fewer binges, and thus an overall healthier weight.

5. *Eat Adequate Calories*

Our culture has devolved to accept a similar myth surrounding caloric intake. We think less is better. We track. We stress. We obsess. We look at a plate as piles of calories, instead of piles of food. We make our choices not based on nutrition, but on a number calculated using a numerical method created in the late nineteenth century that isn't accurate for everyone.

Say you are trying to lose weight and have to choose between two snacks. Pretend, as one *New Scientist* writer did in a story called "The Calorie Delusion: Why Food Labels Are Wrong," that they're a 250-calorie pre-packaged brownie and a 300-calorie muesli bar. You choose the brownie, because we've been brainwashed into believing that calories trump all. But there's a cost to digestion that changes depending on what we eat, and this cost is never reflected in the calorie count. The article argues that between the added chewing and digestion required of the muesli bar and the bonus vitamins and minerals you get eating something filled with heart-healthy nuts and seeds, the muesli is a better choice, despite its extra 50 calories. It has more calories, but it takes the body more calories to eat. It'll also make you feel full much longer and give you what a snack is meant to provide—sustained energy—because it takes the body a while to metabolize it.

Over the long term, the true energy used from a brownie is higher, because its carbohydrates are refined and go straight to the bloodstream. The brownie may have fewer calories, but they all get metabolized quickly. In other words, *metabolizable* energy (the number of calories listed on the package) isn't the same thing as the *metabolized* energy (the amount of energy your particular body uses) of any given food. The number of calories on a label aren't necessarily the same as the calories you use.

Those bacteria I discussed before also have a measurable impact on how we use the calories we ingest; for example, some researchers estimate that they consume up to 25 percent of the dietary fiber calories we take in. A study in *The American Journal of Clinical Nutrition* concluded that how we use calories greatly depends not just on what we eat, but on what foods we eat *together*. Different combinations of carbohydrates, for example, may be processed or excreted based on what we eat with them. So the concept that we all get the same amount of energy out of that bar or brownie is just wrong. Thinking that we all need the same number of calories in a day is just as flawed.

Almost anyone who has tried dieting has tried counting and cutting calories. It's awful. Regular days turn into trials of tallying and plotting and, often, weighing and rejecting foods we used to eat without shame. We spend *hours* calculating each day, entwining our entire self-worth with the number that appears after dinner. We axe calories because we've accepted the conventional wisdom that the less we consume, the less we weigh.

Ironically, it's a flawed approach. Our bodies love stability. Think about the tight regulation of everything a doctor measures; we have specific guidelines for blood pressure, blood sugar, iron levels, you name it. The same is true for weight, so when we do anything that undermines the body's natural weight—like trying to cut calories—the body compensates by decreasing metabolism.

The Typical Dieting Day

Below is an example of the average daily menu my clients report aiming for when they come in for weight loss. They are trying to consume far too little. Usually, after four or five appointments, the truth begins to leak out. Because they're hungry, they often end up overeating late at night or medicating with alcohol. They are so shamed by their diet "failures" that they find themselves perpetually feeling one of two things: hunger or defeat.

- **Breakfast:** Toast with jam or nonfat yogurt
- **Lunch:** Salad with just vegetables (or maybe a small piece of fish or chicken), with fat-free or low-fat dressing
- **Snack:** Piece of fruit
- **Dinner:** Pasta with red sauce and broccoli, or boneless, skinless chicken breast and broccoli

---

From an evolutionary perspective, humans learned to consume less when faced with drought or famine. Still today, when we consume less, we send the body into metabolic panic, causing it to hoard fat out of fear that it needs to prepare for long-term calorie deprivation. In effect, eating less acts as a huge stop sign in our metabolic system, which is exactly the opposite of what we want. (As reported in *The Calorie Myth*, by Jonathan Bailor, studies as far back as World War II showed that restricting caloric intake can actually slow the body's metabolic rate by up to 40 percent.) When we stop eating, our body stops working. If weight loss is your goal, the best thing you can offer your body is stability, in the form of dependable, regular eating.

The typical day of eating for someone who is restricting caloric intake usually results in two things: Either they don't even make it to dinner, because they're starving when they come home from work and need to start eating immediately, or they have dinner and then never stop eating, again because they're so hungry. Typically, once people realize how hungry they are, it's impossible to stop eating. Sound familiar? It's not surprising.

Your body isn't getting what it needs, which results in things like hunger and fatigue. My clients report spending the majority of their after-dinner eating time beating themselves up—they can't stop eating or shaming themselves, which stresses the mind and the body, causing the same sort of fight-or-flight response our ancestors depended on for survival. Our metabolism comes to a screeching halt. Eating makes us feel sated enough to prevent both the stress and hunger that makes diets fail, and also increases metabolism, so our natural body weight changes.

The "calories in, calories out" mentality, which has prevailed since the 1950s, makes it near impossible to wrap one's head around the concept that eating more could actually help us. It's even become a moral issue; stand in line at a latte counter for ten minutes, and you'll see the way people ordering nonfat lattes hold their head higher, while people asking for whole-milk mochas look down or directly at the cash register. Ditto for restaurants. "Would you like dessert tonight, sir?" asks the waiter. "Well, I *shouldn't*, but I will." I waited tables for years, and predictably, women would order salads for dinner, then giggle with their friends, decide to be "bad," and order dessert. We have created a society that shames eating, so many of us simply don't feel comfortable eating in public. Similarly, exercising is considered *being* good instead of doing something that *feels* good. We have learned that consuming calories makes us bad, fat, lazy people and burning calories makes us saintly and thin. Both are wrong.

We can simplify explaining why we need calories by explaining where those calories go. The body is amazing. Under the skin, a wise, intricate, self-governing chemistry set is constantly busy allocating nutrients to all the different systems that comprise the human body. You probably realize that your body needs a certain number of calories just to operate—you know, lungs breathing, heart beating, blood flowing, etcetera. Before we even start placing extra demands on it, in the form of stress, exercise, and daily activities, the body has an awful lot to do. We breathe more than twenty thousand times a day, for example, and that requires calories. So does talking. So does thinking.

But exactly how many calories do we need? Let's make it simple: Assume, as Eileen Stellefson Myers does in *Winning the War Within,* that you're a five-foot-two woman, aged nineteen, who weighs a hundred pounds and does nothing all day long. You don't leave your bed. You don't go for a walk or put groceries away. You don't fetch the mail. Sitting still, with that tiny frame and those tiny muscles and those tiny organs, you burn 1,200 calories a day. Doing nothing.

Where Calories Go

The following is an example of where 1,200 calories go for a five-foot-two, inactive nineteen-year-old who weighs only a hundred pounds.

- **Heart:** 144 calories
- **Kidneys:** 144 calories
- **Liver:** 276 calories
- **Brain:** 276 calories
- **Skeletal muscle:** 360 calories

So what happens if you're taller, thicker, and more active? Most of us are all of those things. Clearly, we need more energy. While the number of calories we each need depends on our frame, metabolism, and activity level, we all need calories and plenty of them. If we don't get them, our less vital organs shut down. Our body prioritizes the most necessary organs—so we keep breathing and beating—but anything that's nonessential gets its resources ripped off. Our thinking falters. Our skin pales. Our fingers get cold. Our hair falls out. And, in an effort to preserve what little energy we have left (especially if we're exercising like crazy in an attempt to lose weight), our body tries to preserve our fat stores. Again, our metabolism slows down.

In other words, fad diets don't work because they starve us of vital nutrients. When we inevitably "break down" and start eating more again—which happens not because we're weak willed, but because the diet isn't

Are You Getting Enough?

Signs that you may not be getting enough calories include:

- Fatigue
- Hunger
- Constant feeling of cold and/or cold hands
- Irritability
- Foggy thinking
- Dizziness when moving from sitting to standing
- Poor concentration
- Difficulty sleeping

physiologically sustainable for us in the long term and the body is smart enough to tell us so—we are relieving our bodies of a period of what is, in effect, starvation. (I often compare calorie restriction to the practice of bloodletting, because I believe eventually we will see it as just as archaic.) My approach isn't magic. It isn't fast, either; finding the body's ideal weight often takes many months. But it is a little miraculous. When we get enough calories, eventually, our body relaxes. Our fight-or-flight response subsides, and our hormones self-regulate. **That's the metabolism miracle: the body burns more calories and operates more efficiently—resulting in more energy, increased immunity, more lustrous skin and hair, a healthier gut, and better moods—when we simply eat enough real food.**

6. Eat Regularly

If you've tried multiple diets and felt the disappointment that comes when you can't stick with one, you've likely also experienced the cycle of self-promise and self-hate that comes with what the most recent diet defines as overeating. It works like this: You follow the diet all day long. You eat a "sensible" dinner. Before bed, you open the fridge and have a yogurt, because you want just a little something more, but you don't want anything too fattening. You eat it standing up. You're still hungry. You have a handful of walnuts and a cup of applesauce, but still no go. You open the chocolate chips. Suddenly, it's the Last Supper again, and because tomorrow is a new day and you promise, promise, promise it will be different, you decide, possibly while crying, that you need ice cream next. You go to bed exhausted and sad but finally full, and in the morning, because of the previous night, you eat just an apple for breakfast. Or no breakfast at all. You think you're doing even better than the diet demands for the morning, but after dinner, the same thing happens. You're not getting enough.

No matter how much we've eaten the previous day, we still need calories to function. Eating regularly—morning, noon, and night, and usually a few times in between—establishes a dependable stream of metabolism-boosting hormones, which prevent us from overeating and help us think more clearly and sleep better. (I've worked with a lot of body builders who keep food

My Story: Eating Enough

It may sound strange, but because of the way I grew up, I'm good at starving. I spent so much of my childhood hungry that I often don't realize I need food until the physical signs show up. (I shake, and my head starts feeling thick, and I start snapping at people. When I finally eat, I eat like an NFL player. It's not pretty.) But like many of my long-term clients, I can tell I haven't been eating enough in general when I start gaining weight. It sounds crazy, I know, but it's true; restricting calories is an easy, predictable way for me to grow out of my jeans.

To ward off the effects of "hanger," as the dangerous combination of hunger and anger is sometimes known, I recommend clients practice preventative eating. In the short term, scheduling snacks that contain both fat and protein—calories!—keep my moods and energy even. In the long term, they keep me from having to buy new clothes when I get busy. I usually carry a bag with water, nuts or cheese, vegetables, and kefir or cottage cheese with me most of the time. I keep nuts and canned fish in my car for emergency situations. (I think of it as the grown-up version of the box of Cheerios many parents keep in their cars for screaming toddlers.) I even keep food by the bed, which for many seems like a cardinal sin.

by the bed and set an alarm for the middle of the night so they can eat to keep their metabolism strong. I wouldn't recommend this, but I think it illustrates the point.)

In *The Slow Down Diet*, Marc David explains how metabolism actually changes throughout the day, getting faster as the sun comes up and slower as the sun goes down, with the peak at midday. In the United States, we tend to eat our big meal at night, whereas in many cultures, lunch is the largest spread. From a scientific perspective, it makes much more sense to stretch our consumption out throughout a day, rather than save it up for the evening, right before we go to bed, when our metabolism is at its lowest. Like nutrition pioneer Adelle Davis recommended, eat breakfast like a king, lunch like a prince, and dinner like a pauper.

Eating regularly also specifically supports the adrenal glands. The adrenals—two walnut-size glands sitting nonchalantly on top of the kidneys, where you've probably never noticed them—play a crucial role in producing estrogen and stress hormones such as cortisol. In addition to helping us manage stress, the hormones help us regulate moods, digestion, inflammation, and hunger. They're efficient if we eat consistently throughout the day.

If we're highly stressed, though, or don't eat regularly enough, they get tired and overworked. When the adrenals stop producing hormones, the body begins relying on fat cells, which produce the same hormones in much smaller quantities. As a result, the body begins holding on to fat in an attempt to preserve hormonal balance, which often translates to fatty deposits around the abdomen. (This is particularly true in women around and after the age of menopause, when estrogen production also slows in the ovaries. Sound familiar? It's the body's normal, natural reaction to low hormone levels.) However, when we eat regularly—and especially when we eat meals sitting down, without the added stress of distractions such as work and television—we become calmer and eat less. As a result, we are less stressed, and our adrenal glands function better. If you're in the habit of eating on the go and/or eating at wildly erratic times, you'll likely notice weight loss if you begin eating more regularly in a calm environment. Many people find breakfast and lunch the most difficult meals to consume regularly. If this is you, consider packing a lunch box the night before, so that even if you're on the go, you're at least eating, and if you can find a break to eat, you're well prepared.

7. Accept the Metabolism Miracle

I can hear you. *Calories. How can it* not *be about calories?* That the best approach to reliable, long-term weight loss is regular, adequate caloric intake is really difficult for most lifetime dieters to grasp. And that's not surprising. Living life a certain way creates habits—and having those habits backed up by two generations of oversimplified conventional wisdom makes them really, really hard to break.

Over and over again, you've heard from others (but more importantly, from yourself) that you've failed to lose weight because you lack willpower. Because you simply ate too many calories. You've somehow learned to live with the oppressive shadow of the shame associated with eating, which, theoretically, we are all supposed to do. Yet, you also intrinsically know that counting calories doesn't work. You don't want just another short-term solution. Comparing calories in with calories out is an oversimplified view of an infinitely complex equation. You know because you've tried, over and over, and every time you restrict calories, your weight goes down, only to yo-yo right back up again, often higher than before. You're reading this because you're looking for something different. Know this: The diets don't fail because of you. The diets fail because the diets themselves are flawed. They confuse the body, thereby causing it to hold on to weight because it can't trust *us* to regulate our own eating.

The diets are also quite dated. That eating low fat (and by extension, low calorie) is a trend that started in the 1950s is something we often overlook. Since then, the science has changed dramatically. How many of us still use computers that fill entire rooms, rotary-dial telephones that are still connected to a physical telephone line, and cars with carburetors? Precious few. If you want to be a weight-loss hipster, go for it. Follow the vintage science. But don't forget that the mind-set most Americans follow when they want to lose weight emerged when Eisenhower was president, and since then, our national health has plummeted. (In 2009, the United States ranked fiftieth worldwide in terms of life expectancy, behind Bosnia and South Korea.) For most of us, accepting the metabolism miracle, which holds that eating will change our metabolism for the *better*, is the best, most sustainable path to weight loss.

You've noted, I'm sure, that I still haven't told you how *much* to eat. And I'm not going to. That's your job. With my clients, I only start addressing portion sizes and emotional eating once they've given themselves permission to eat and have started focusing on whole foods, good fats and proteins, and bacteria-rich foods. However, I can help you learn to do your job. In fact, that's my favorite part of *my* job. In Chapter 8, I'll start teaching you how to listen to your body. First, though, I'll talk about the foods I find miraculous.

....

THE PRESCRIPTION

- Understand that calories in versus calories out isn't an accurate or appropriate way to approach weight loss.
- Address and set yourself free of feelings of failure.
- Follow the Seven Steps to Weight Loss.
- Accept the Metabolism Miracle.

Chapter 7

FOOD MIRACLES, BODY MIRACLES

Many people are alive but don't touch
the miracle of being alive.

—Thich Nhat Hanh

In her late fifties, Jill came into Passionate Nutrition after hearing me speak on the radio. She went through a lot of tissues during that first appointment as she explained to me that doctors frequently blamed her ailments on aging. She had such low energy that it was hard for her to get through life's day-to-day requirements. She had gone to appointment after appointment with no real response from her doctors—no diagnosis, no results, and certainly no hope. She'd almost accepted that it was just her lot in life to age painfully.

I told her I don't buy how our culture blames any mystery illness on aging. I said that if she and I were hiking in the Swiss Alps, we would be getting passed by eighty-year-olds. If we were in India, we'd be getting schooled by ninety-year-old matriarchs. As we talked, her actions and stories made it clear to me that she was exceptionally depleted even though she shopped at co-ops. She was getting by on easy-to-grab foods that weren't nutrient dense; years of eating this way had left her weak and feeling powerless. Right away, we focused on getting nutrient-rich foods (such as nettles and seaweed) and power-packed proteins (red meat and sardines among them) into her diet to rebuild her system. The results, though not instantaneous, were extraordinary. Her energy improved dramatically, which changed her life on many levels. She felt like a new woman—she felt *younger*.

As humans—people who spend a lot of time sitting on the couch feeling lousy because our energy is low, our joints hurt, or we're just too ashamed of ourselves to do anything else—we are easily tricked into thinking the latest fad diet will change things. We know, though, that every time we try a new diet, we tend to fail. But listen big, people: Your poor health is not necessarily the result of what you're eating. The cause is likely what you're *not* eating.

This chapter doesn't contain tips. Instead it describes the *requirements* for a healthy life. **If you finish this book having retained one thing—that adding the foods described in this next section, such as seaweed and shellfish, can change your life—then I'll consider myself a success.** If you want to transform your health, consider this chapter your manifesto.

The Seven Food Miracles

A lot of us know that colorful foods have more nutrients. Dark vegetables such as sweet or purple potatoes, beets, kale, and spinach are high in antioxidants; potatoes are high in potassium; and broccoli is packed with vitamin C. But what we often don't realize—and what I specialize in, after spending years living completely off the grid in Colorado and on the Washington coast—is that vegetables that grow in the sea and in the wild often have tenfold the vitamins and nutrients of farmed vegetables. On a nutritional scale, comparing kale, the powerhouse darling of the nutrient world, to seaweed is like comparing iceberg lettuce to kale. Seaweed kicks kale's butt. The same applies to nettles. (For example, 1 cup of kale contains 206 milligrams of calcium, which is one of its big claims to fame, but 1 cup of dried nettles, which is about a big handful, has 2,900 milligrams.) I'm not asking you to crawl into the woods to eat only nettles and seaweed and never come out. I just want you to open your eyes to the food available in our own backyards, often quite literally.

The Seven Food Miracles

- Seaweed
- Foraged food
- Shellfish
- Sardines
- Red meat
- Organ meats
- Fermented foods

Eating wild foods means looking to food sources that haven't been tampered with much over the course of human history. They range from ocean foods such as fish, shellfish, and seaweed—because we haven't harnessed and changed entire oceans quite yet, those foods retain their original mineral-rich benefits—to such foraged foods as nettles, dandelion, and mushrooms. Wild foods are also those with ingredients humans don't totally control, such as grass-fed beef from cows who are allowed to choose what they eat, and fermented foods, whose beneficial bacteria grow and thrive without our intervention.

Although the list is miles long and there are runners-up like wild mushrooms and roots, I've narrowed the world of wild foods down to seven "miracles." They're not miracles in the sense that they can cure cancer or stop painful inflammation the second you swallow them. They're miracles because they still provide all the nutrition food is inherently supposed to contain. And when we get good nutrition, the scary things—the cancers, the inflammation—often aren't as villainous. Food has the power to heal in ways medicine never will. Once you understand how certain foods can expand your nutritional repertoire (and generate a little creativity in the kitchen, to boot), I'll move on to the real miracle: the human body.

1. Seaweed

Although it may not be something you're used to eating, seaweed consumption is by no means new. Seaweed has anchored the Japanese diet for millennia. The Maya used a gel made with sea moss to make desserts. Maritime cultures worldwide have learned that because it can be enjoyed raw or dried, and because it grows absurdly quickly in the summertime and stores amazingly well, seaweed is a good, reliable dietary staple. It's no accident that farmers have learned kelp makes an effective crop fertilizer; its nutrients make things grow. Even when we eat it in just small amounts, those benefits extend to us. Seaweed can nourish the thyroid, promote digestive movement, help prevent cancer, and make skin and hair more luminous.

Seaweed is also a strong detoxifier. In a world where exposure to radioactive and chemical waste can be more frequent than we might wish, a quickly renewable food source capable of removing mercury, cadmium, lead, barium, tin, and other heavy metals from our bodies is a miracle indeed. That the removal of harmful toxins comes with a dose of the minerals we rely on for daily function is an excellent bonus—seaweed is nourished by the ocean, which contains salts and minerals in the same proportion as they are found in human blood. Depending on the variety, dried seaweed can contain up to 50 percent minerals, which means it beats any land-grown vegetable every time as a source of essentials such as potassium, calcium, magnesium, zinc, copper, sulfur, selenium, bromine, iodine, and iron, to name a few. Plus, it tastes good.

From a dietary perspective, eating foods that contain seaweed or adding seaweed to foods you normally cook (think burger patties or spaghetti sauce), equates to an easy insurance program. Regular intake gives the body the nutrients it needs for cell health. From a cosmetic perspective, this translates to radiant skin, but inside, it means stronger digestion, lower inflammation, and better immune function. Start with mild-flavored seaweed such as arame, which can be added to salad, or with dulse, which comes in powdered form and can be sprinkled into soups, salads, or sauces (often without affecting the flavor of whatever you're eating). I add a strip of kombu to anything I cook in water—beans or grains, for example.

At home, I lead seaweed harvesting and drying seminars, so I almost always have many varieties of dried seaweed on hand, but I understand that's not the norm in most kitchen cupboards. Many large supermarkets (and definitely most natural food stores) carry a variety of seaweeds from reliable sources.

Seaweed for Beginners

Different types of seaweed contain different nutrient levels; some have more calcium, for example, while others have more iron. But overall, seaweed has the broadest nutrient range of any vegetable. A little goes a long way. It's better to eat just a little bit every day than to eat a seaweed salad once a week. As a general guideline, think about adding ½ to 1 teaspoon of powdered seaweed or 1 to 3 tablespoons of dried seaweed to an entire dish. The goal is to enhance the flavor of the food, not turn your birthday cake into a seaweed cake.

---

2. Foraged Food

Sure, broccoli's good for you. So are turnip greens, kale, spinach, and asparagus. I usually tell my clients to aim for making up half of their plate with vegetables. But it's a little oversimplified to just say that green stuff is good for you, because, like meats and dairy, not all greens are created equal. Think of a food's power the way you think of a person's upbringing; someone who has been coddled and pampered often has fewer life skills, less self-esteem, and a weaker personality than someone who has survived great trials. I'm a good example; I had a hell of a childhood, but today, having persevered and fought for (sometimes literal) survival, I'm a hearty, robust, tenacious person. Food is the same way; a food's suffering leads to its strength. Organic vegetables, for example, have more antioxidants because they're not artificially protected by pesticides. If you buy the market's twistiest, turniest vegetables—the ones that have suffered and fought on their way to maturity—you're buying better nutrition.

It took me a long time to internalize that a plant's properties aren't there purely for human benefit; plants have vitamins and minerals because they need them to survive. Perhaps you've heard that garlic is more beneficial to the body if you let it sit for a bit after chopping it. You're letting it sit because the plant, in a last-ditch effort to survive, is undergoing an enzymatic reaction that strengthens how its antioxidants act inside the body. It's stronger because it's trying to stay alive. We get more benefit because it's been beaten up.

Food that has worked hard to thrive by bending around rocks, saving water, fighting off predator plants, and digging its roots deep, deep into the ground contains more of the nutrients we need. Foraged burdock will have more nutrients than farm-raised burdock, just like wild berries will be better for you (and often tastier!) than their farm-grown cousins. Foraged in the wild, edibles such as stinging nettle, dandelion leaves and root, cleavers, burdock, chickweed, raspberry leaf, rose hips, oat straw, and comfrey, to name just a few of the things I forage myself near my own home, are all excellent sources of the vitamins and minerals we work so hard to eat. We could learn a lot from them; many are ancient herbs that have survived for millennia by being, in a word, tough. They also grow in soil that, unlike land used to grow many grocery store foods, hasn't been depleted of the nutrients we need.

Harvesting wild food is not a practice for the weak or fastidious. When I lived off the grid, I spent a lot of time digging, and often got really, really dirty. (Dirt and the microorganisms it contains are also good for digestion, so while I don't eat the clumps of mud in my cilantro, I should note that I rarely wash my vegetables. Many of the fragile vitamins exist in their most exterior layer, and can be harmed or sloughed right off by an aggressive scrub brush.) However, today, many of the foods I find regularly in the wild are available in dried form at natural foods stores or fresh at farmers' markets. Ask around—many farmers have small amounts of wild edibles such as purslane, miner's lettuce, mushrooms, and whatever else happens to grown nearby. And ask them how they eat their wild greens. Most can just be torn and added to salads or soups, which is my favorite way to incorporate them. Some, like stinging nettles, need to be cooked or dried before you eat them. (Stinging nettles come by their name honestly, but cooking or drying them causes the fine, stinging hairs on the sunny side of each leaf to calm down and become completely harmless.)

For general health, think of foraged greens as nature's supplements. Susun Weed, the herbalist behind the Wise Woman Herbal book series, taught me about infusions and has written extensively on the topic. For an easy way to start, see the Nettle Infusion recipe (page 219). Even better, sign up for a foraging class and learn how to enjoy the benefits of the plants in your own backyard.

3. *Shellfish*

When clients come in with extreme fatigue, lack of appetite, unexpected weight gain, anemia, or depression—and often with more than one of these, since they're frequently related—I send them to the fishmonger. Shellfish such as oysters, mussels, and clams are an excellent source of vitamin B_{12}, which helps keep our blood cells healthy. In addition, shellfish have very high levels of zinc, the mineral that, as I'll discuss in Chapter 9, offers major skin health benefits. To put it in perspective, zinc is such a common deficiency that I assume people are zinc-deficient unless proven otherwise. We use zinc in our immune systems, where it inhibits virus production and viral RNA synthesis, and in thyroid and sex hormone regulation. (Almost nothing compares to the zinc level in an oyster, raw or cooked, which is one reason I feel so lucky to live in Washington State.) Shellfish have high levels of L-tryptophan, the mood-regulating and calming amino acid that we use to make serotonin. Like grass-fed beef, they also contain essential fatty acids and saturated fat, which is key to satiety and skin and brain health.

4. Sardines

In *The Jungle Effect*, a historical exploration of foods around the world, physician and anthropological historian Daphne Miller makes a convincing argument that the world's healthiest cultures—those with the lowest incidences of heart disease, diabetes, and depression—all eat sardines or similar little fish. Likewise, when I was abroad, I noticed that from Japan and China to Europe to the coast of Africa to Central America, families relied on small, oily fish as a dietary staple far more than we do in the United States. Until I started traveling, I'd never heard of them. Once I tried them, I was hooked.

The Doctrine of Signatures

Frequently, Passionate Nutrition's specific recommendations match the Doctrine of Signatures, a sixteenth-century theory that states that the foods and herbs best for certain body parts look a lot like those body parts. Bone broth is good for bones, kidney beans help heal kidneys, walnuts can improve brain health, and carrots (think of them sliced into rounds) help with vision. Interestingly, peanuts, which are often associated with male libido, were often banned by churches in the Middle Ages. Not surprisingly, one of the main ingredients in Viagra is derived from—you guessed it—peanuts. The Doctrine of Signatures may seem hokey today, but know that much of the common knowledge we accept has roots in this Renaissance practice. Oysters, for example, have a thick, viscous liquid thought to resemble sperm, and were thus used as an aphrodisiac, which is why we consider them a "romantic" food today. They also look similar to a vagina inside. (It also happens that shellfish are rich in zinc, which has been shown to increase sex drive.)

For a while, I had a reputation in the nutrition community as "Sardine Girl." A new client once sat in my office for her first appointment, then called me on it at the end of our session. "Wait, aren't you going to tell me to eat more sardines?" she asked. My reputation had preceded me.

But she was right. I did tell her to eat more sardines, because if I were to choose only one "miracle" food, it might be this tiny, oil-rich fish found along almost every coastline. They're as delicious canned as they are fresh (actually, more so, if you ask me). They're perfect for snacking, and even kids often like them on crackers. Salmon are known for omega-3s, the essential fatty acids the body depends on for everything from reducing inflammation to immune function to retinal health. Sardines actually have higher levels of EFAs than salmon. (Since they're smaller fish, they also bio-accumulate fewer toxic heavy metals, such as mercury, than large fish.) I tell clients to take advantage of them because they're significantly cheaper and more convenient to eat.

Eating sardines doesn't require befriending a fishmonger or learning how to cook them the way fancy chefs do. (Incidentally, they're very easy to cook; just slather them in oil and sear or grill them for a few minutes on each side over medium-high heat.) Treat tinned sardines the way you would tuna fish; use them in sandwiches and salads, blended with sour cream or mayonnaise for a powerful morning or afternoon snack. I personally love mixing them with sour cream, salt, and a big handful of chopped tarragon.

5. *Red Meat*

The saturated fat and essential fatty acids found in red meat contribute to the structural integrity of our cells and strengthen muscle tissues. (We will talk more about the benefits of fats in Chapter 9.) More specifically, though, red meat also contains cholesterol, which plays a part in every detail of our body's functioning.

Every animal on the planet makes cholesterol. It makes up almost half the membrane of every cell in the human body, both as a result of our food, and thanks to the liver, the cholesterol factory inside each and every person.

Yet we've labeled cholesterol as the big bad wolf lurking inside much of what we eat, even though its main job is exactly that—to lurk inside us, and help us *use* what we eat.

Cholesterol is not the enemy. Really, we should be thankful it's there. Cholesterol is behind the synapses that form memories, the regulation of all human sex hormones, and the proper function of the entire immune system. As such, cholesterol-lowering drugs often cause memory loss, infertility or decreases in virility, and impaired immunity. Research shows that quality of life and longevity can actually improve with higher cholesterol levels. An extensive study in the journal *Neurology* showed that elderly people with the *highest* cholesterol have 70 percent less chance of suffering from dementia; Japanese researchers linked very low cholesterol levels with higher morbidity rates. Likewise, in 2013, a paper in the *Journal of American Medical Directors Association* concluded that cholesterol levels were *unrelated* to mortality in subjects between the ages of seventy and ninety.

I've personally experienced a need for cholesterol in my diet too. After thirteen years of hard-core vegetarianism, when I was also experimenting with veganism, my cholesterol was at its highest. Doctors chastised me about my diet and got angry when I refused to take cholesterol-lowering medications. Later, I found out hypothyroidism was causing my high cholesterol; today, I eat loads of butter, cream, and eggs, yet my cholesterol is in what modern doctors would consider a "safe" zone. Most of my clients find the same thing happens; eating more cholesterol in whole foods, not less, tends to change their lab results, which pleases their general practitioners.

However, I'm not saying you should ignore your cholesterol levels; in fact, cholesterol makes for a really good messenger because it tells us about our body's woes. One of cholesterol's key roles is preventing disease and healing wounds, so high levels mean the body is fighting something, and fighting hard. In my case, my body was battling a thyroid problem. I needed to pay more attention to my thyroid (by feeding it shellfish, seaweed, and nettles), not the data that worried the doctor. Cholesterol is the body's tattletale;

rather than focus on our high cholesterol numbers, we should try to determine exactly what real problem all that cholesterol is trying to flag.

Advocating that people "eat more red meat" is sort of misleading. I personally love the grounding, satisfying effect red meat has on me. I like its texture, and that it's easy to cook. But ultimately, it's what red meat offers—satiety, great flavor, clear thinking, and a *healthy* dose of saturated fat and cholesterol—that I'm after. It also offers iron, the nutrient that makes the meat red and one of the most prevalent nutrient deficiencies worldwide, especially among women, and zinc, which most Americans are deficient in. Learn to relabel red meat as something your body needs and loves.

6. *Organ Meats*

Watch any energetic cat eat an animal he brings into a house, and you'll notice a trend: like his big-cat cousins (and, in fact, most natural predators), he'll tear his prey open and eat its organs first. Fluffy isn't trying to gross you out. He's doing what no mama cat ever had to teach him, going for the guts first because organs are the most nutritious parts of the animals we eat. Wander the African savannah, and you'll notice that many carcasses still have much of their meat attached but the insides are always eaten clean.

Humans have a strong history of eating organs too. Hearts, livers, kidneys, and sweetbreads aren't just common to many global cuisines; they're central to them. For example, Native Americans, like many Eastern cultures, have long believed that eating certain organs benefits the associated organs in humans. Eating hearts benefits your heart; eating kidneys benefits your kidneys. But in the United States, we've grown unaccustomed to eating anything but animal muscle, which means we miss out on the vitamins, minerals, and amino acids that organ meats offer in generous quantities.

But it's not just those vitamins and minerals that are important. It's how they react inside your body that matters. Specifically, offal, as organ meats are sometimes called, contains the right ratio of nutrients and fat for your body to use all of them appropriately. Liver, for example, is widely considered nature's best source of vitamin A, a fat-soluble vitamin that helps with hormone, immune, and digestive function. Beta-carotene, a precursor to vitamin A, is available in plants high in carotenoids, such as carrots, but we require fat to process vitamin A, which carrots don't have. That's why we only absorb 39 percent of carrots' beta-carotene (and that's only when they're cooked in fat). When we eat liver, we get vitamin A along with the fat it requires for absorption, so we actually use that vitamin A to its greatest effect. Similarly, iron, which meat contains in large quantities, is more bioavailable in organ meats, as are vitamins D and K (which are often difficult to absorb from supplements), because offal offers all the tools for digesting them in the same bite.

That eating an animal's internal organs increases the sustainability of farming in general (because you're not wasting valuable, edible parts) is an awfully nice side effect. As always, try to buy organic, pastured animals whenever you can. You can learn to cook the organs individually, but it's often quite easy to find sausages and pâtés that celebrate the whole beast. At home, I buy ground organ meats from the farmers' market and mix them into burgers, tacos, chili, enchiladas, and meat loaf. The kids have no idea.

7. *Fermented Foods*

Although I discussed how fermented foods form the foundation of gut health in Chapter 4, it's worth reiterating here just how powerful they can be. In his best-selling book *The Art of Fermentation*, expert Sandor Ellix Katz explains how fermented foods invigorate and strengthen the immune system. I've found that my clients are often astonished by how much their winters change after they start eating fermented foods; they no longer fall prey to the same flus and colds that used to render them helpless two or three times every year. Recent research has also showed prebiotics and pro-biotics can help prevent colon cancer and spur weight loss; one European study linked milk fermented with just one strain of bacteria with a 5 percent decrease in abdominal fat after just twelve weeks of regular consumption.

Fermented foods go well beyond the "Fab Five" discussed in Chapter 4. From homemade uncanned pickles to cultured sour cream and cultured butter, healthy doses of beneficial bacteria are available in different forms of the foods you probably already eat—think raw cheeses, cultured cottage cheese, and yogurt. (Beer, wine, and cider are fermented foods as well and have the same benefits if you can buy them unpasteurized.) Make fermented foods staples of your everyday diet.

The Miracle of the Human Body

Instead of defining certain foods as miraculous, perhaps we should think of factory-produced foods as predators. Many people who find they're sensitive to wheat products, for example, can eat things made with spelt, the precursor to the modern wheat plant, or they can eat sprouted-grain bread. Spelt isn't a miracle grain; it's simply less harmful than something more processed. Similarly, sprouted grains are easier to digest than today's genetically "advanced" grains. Every month, I watch clients who identify as lactose intolerant learn they can eat dairy products if they're fermented. (It's no accident that so many people who can't drink milk can still drink kefir and traditionally made yogurt.) Kefir isn't necessarily a miracle, it's just that fermenting milk breaks down its sugars and lactose, making it easier to digest.

The true miracle is the human body. Frankly, I think we all lack the awe and respect we owe our own spiritual and physical homes. I've spent a decade and a half working with clients who have made a habit of assaulting their bodies—bulimic and anorexic clients who have rejected all caloric intake; poisoned clients like myself who spent years subsisting solely on what amounts to processed wheat, sugar, and toxins; well-meaning clients who deprive their bodies of the fat required for survival in an attempt to fit societal ideals. Still, we survive. Despite that we've learned to abuse ourselves, our bodies are resilient. While we seem to think, on a cultural level, that we have total control over the body, its innate wisdom rules. If we drink too much, the liver regenerates. If we need calcium desperately, the body can actually transform silica (found in oats, millet, barley, potatoes, wheat, and wild foods like horsetail) into calcium for us. This transformational ability, known as biological transmutation, has changed my view of the world of nutrition.

The miracle is that, no matter what's happened in the past, we have the tools we need to heal and thrive in the future. We have our own bodies.

Our Changeable Genetic Code

One client came to me after years of battling weight. Starting as a teenager, she'd tried a plethora of different diets, always eventually bouncing back to (or above) her previous weight. By age twenty, she'd all but given up hope. She'd grown up in a family of overweight people who relied heavily on processed foods and felt sentenced to a lifetime of depression and anxiety surrounding eating. She had skin problems, constant fatigue, acid reflux, heavy-metal toxicity, and hosted a revolving door of random infections.

Working with us to change her diet over the course of almost a decade, she lost more than a hundred pounds. But for her, the real miracle occurred when she realized she had changed the way her body functioned overall. She'd always just assumed she was programmed to be unhealthy, but over that decade, the slow, steady march toward health had shown her body a different path. She will never have the body we see in magazines, but she found what was healthy for her body type. Today, although she focuses on incorporating healthful foods into her diet, she is also much more flexible about what she eats and has a much more joyful relationship with food.

Her story isn't unusual in my practice. People walk in all the time with little to no expectation that they can change how their bodies operate. But it's not a pipe dream; the miracle of the body is that it changes. Because no cell in the human body lasts a lifetime, we are constantly morphing into new versions of ourselves. That paper cut you got last week when you were opening bills? It's probably gone, because we regenerate the skin on our entire body every seven days. (That's upwards of thirty thousand skin cells each minute!)

With only a few exceptions, the entire body is replaced every seven years, which means we have the opportunity to repair tissues and change cellular habits, even as we get older. Changing eating habits allows us to renew ourselves and reverse what we previously viewed as lifelong sentences to being overweight or unhealthy in some specific way. Damaged skin cells become healthy, more radiant skin cells. Tired muscles become more energetic muscles. Ineffective, painful digestion becomes smooth, pain-free digestion. Crippled hormones become better, happier, more effective hormones. Destroyed immune function becomes strong immune function. You become a new you, top to bottom, inside and out.

We aren't sentenced to the genetic ailments of our pasts, either. Studies show that negative or positive thoughts can actually affect how our DNA expresses itself. Lissa Rankin, a doctor and the author of *Mind Over Medicine*, explains that just as the placebo effect can help us heal, a "nocebo" effect, as she calls the belief some hold that they're fated to suffer certain medical ailments, can actually cause those very ailments.

Neuroscientist Jerre Levy offers an excellent analogy that explains we aren't all destined to be any or all of the things our relatives are or have been. Genes are like library books, she says, meaning that most of them stay on the shelves and get dusty. While the body "checks out" many genes, like those that give us our mother's nose or our father's thick hair, many of the genes we carry are never expressed. Most undesirable genetic expressions—genes that may be related to cancers, inflammation, or other negative conditions—only surface under the influence of an environmental condition, such as stress, fatigue, pollution, or poor nutrition. Staying mindful of those conditions keeps the genes on the shelves, so to speak. Miraculous, indeed.

A Positive Change

Enjoying food actually allows us to get more of what we need from it. As reported by Marc David, founder of the Institute for the Psychology of Eating, a group of Thai and Swedish researchers proved that the body digests and assimilates more nutrients from food when we actually enjoy what we're eating. In the study, Thai subjects absorbed more nutrients from a Thai diet, which they enjoyed, than from a Swedish diet, which they reported not enjoying as much; the reverse was true of Swedish subjects. In other words, our mental state has a lot to do with how we absorb the food we eat.

David argues (and I agree) that when food tastes good to us, it does more for the body than when we don't like it. Making your food taste good—and allowing yourself to really enjoy it—allows you to absorb nutrients more effectively, which leads to a better, more energetic you. The opposite goes for feelings such as guilt, shame, anger, and embarrassment, which often plague us when we're eating foods we've designated as "bad" or "forbidden." When we eat with shame, we digest the attitude that we're stuck with poor health, our body sags with the negativity, and we don't absorb nutrients as well. Over the years, I've noticed that for most people, the Seven Food Miracles, in addition to the great benefits described above, are also just intensely enjoyable.

Most of my colleagues sell nutritional supplements to offset the costs of running a nutrition business. I don't. Passionate Nutrition survives and thrives because we teach people how to change their health on a sustainable basis long after any supplement bottle runs out. And our counseling is 100 percent food-based.

I originally named my practice Realize Health because I think the change that comes with this realization—that we really *can* be healthy when we eat differently—is hugely powerful, both physically and mentally. The next time you sit down to a meal (and the next time, and the time after that), do your best to think of the foods on your plate as your allies. Think of them as your saviors. Think of them as the things that, over time, will help that wise body of yours figure out how to heal. Trust that no matter what you've been through, and no matter how many times you've tried to heal in the past, using food as medicine will work. You will realize health.

....

THE PRESCRIPTION

- Incorporate the Seven Food Miracles into your diet.
- Look beyond the grocery store for your food.
- Trust that your body has the power to transform and regenerate.
- Eat abundantly, enjoyably, and positively.

Part III

THE ESSENTIALS

Chapter 8

WHAT IS YOUR BODY SAYING?

*The curious paradox is that when I accept
myself just as I am, then I can change.*

—Carl Rogers

As a society, America is addicted to weight loss. And not surprisingly, the process of trying to lose weight or improve health is in many ways similar to the process addicts go through. Say you're unhappy with your weight. (The same stages apply if you have a debilitating digestive disorder, like I did, or even if you have arthritis that affects how you function each day.) First, you're in denial. You make jokes. You wear huge sweaters until it's eighty degrees outside and avoid any activity that might force you to show your body. Next comes anger. You fight with your significant other about your weight, yell at your kids for no reason, and start to feel hateful emotions toward food. (Remember that old TV show *Roseanne*? It's her.) The refrigerator becomes an enemy. Third, you go into bargaining mode. You make plans to diet, but because it hasn't started yet, you enjoy a last week (or six) of freedom. Depression comes next; it's during this phase, when you might even isolate yourself, that you begin to really seriously overeat or binge. Some people go for ice cream or peanut butter, and some soothe themselves with alcohol, which often leads to even more bingeing. The final stage is acceptance. It's the hardest stage to find, but it's the most important one.

Most of my clients come in ready for change. On the diet front, they've tried them all. If they have a physical malady, they've been to six or eight doctors already. They *need* change. But, perhaps surprisingly, the crux of my work isn't teaching people what to eat. It's teaching people to change their relationships with food and with themselves. It's finding that final stage. For so many of us, eating—and all it entails, like grocery shopping, keeping food in the house, and opening a new jar of peanut butter—can be downright terrifying. We've learned to connect food with shame, guilt, and embarrassment, or simply with pain and sadness. The fear of being sick or feeling fat is often so deeply lodged within our psyche that we have to literally retrain ourselves how to listen to our bodies. In many ways, we have become addicted to feeling bad about ourselves.

After around six months, I tend to slow down and take a look at the habits that bring a client to me in the first place. I'm ready to go deeper, and I often start by helping people recognize how they perceive themselves. *Hello, my name is Angela, and I'm addicted to feeling bad about myself.* This is where nutrition education stops and nutritional counseling begins. It's this process, one of slowing down and learning to be very, very clear about what we want our lives to look like ten or twenty years down the road, that often results in sustainable long-term health, self-acceptance, self-love, and weight loss. It's also a crucial step to go through in order to remove the fear, guilt, and shame associated with eating certain "forbidden" foods. And it starts with recognizing why many of us want to lose weight in the first place.

An Informal History of Dieting

If you follow an anthropologist into ancient caves, you might notice there are no crude sketches of early humans counting calories. There are drawings of hunters chasing big, mangy beasts, and of the kill and the feast that follows. Throughout history, while other species developed fancy feathers or a fabulous mane to lure mates, humans have learned to judge each other's health—and thus their attractiveness—on their ability to take that feast with them in the form of body fat. Until very recently in our evolution, only a woman of a certain size was thought to be strong enough to carry on the family's genes. Thin men and women alike were considered frail, sickly, and unattractive.

Our obsession with size began in earnest at the turn of the last century. Most historians agree there were multiple factors, including, of all things, industrialization. Before then, dresses were tailor-made, but the advent of machinery and mass production meant women became more aware of dress sizes. Around the same time, there was large-scale acceptance of the use of the calorie as a unit of food-energy measurement, and Lulu Hunt Peters, a California doctor, is credited with popularizing the idea of calorie restriction. Although diets meant to help subscribers lose weight—as opposed to eating new or different foods to feel better—started surfacing in the nineteenth century, it wasn't until the early twentieth century that a full-fledged national interest in being thinner took hold.

But many argue that there's a strong historical link between woman's desire to be smaller and man's desire to make her smaller, both physically and politically. Weight has long been associated with power; that the kings of yore were historically quite large is no accident. Some feminists and size historians postulate, and I agree, that the flapper movement of the 1920s, which popularized a rail-thin body ideal for women, was inspired in part by an attempt to prevent women from becoming too powerful as they began voting and their roles in politics expanded.

As women became again less politically powerful in the 1940s and '50s, the curves came back. As late as the early '60s, ads for "Wate-On," a series of popular weight-*gain* products, used actresses like Raquel Welch to advertise their plumping properties. "True beauty includes a full figure," they declared. Curves were considered crucial to attractiveness. (Imagine how different the world might be today if teenagers saw weight-gain pills in the pages of *Vogue*.) That the sexiness of skinny resurged in the tumultuous late 1960s is no surprise to Naomi Wolf, a political activist and author of the best-seller *The Beauty Myth*, who calls dieting "the most potent political sedative in women's history." I see my work as a hugely feminist issue; helping women eat better allows them to think more clearly because they're fed and no longer focusing exclusively on food. (Studies by Dan Reiff, a Washington State psychologist, show that people with disordered eating spend 20 to 65 percent of their waking hours thinking about food, compared with 10 to 15 percent of the time for people with normal eating habits.) A full belly means a happy, powerful, *available* brain. A woman at her natural weight is the best version of herself.

Today, only half a century later, things have changed even more. Women half the size of healthy adorn magazine pages, advertising anorexia like it's the free "gift" you receive when you buy a thousand-dollar handbag. On the biggest American cultural scale, thin is in. Our biological instinct to want to look better still exists, yet now our society tends to link "better" with "thinner," with no floor to the trend. (Note that while eating issues exist elsewhere, many cultures still embrace a voluptuous woman's body as the ideal form.) I agree that as a whole, our bodies have changed with the times; clearly the threats to modern-day humanity are much different than those of a hundred years ago, much less a thousand or more. As a species, we probably don't need to store fat against a drop in the food supply because of a drought or hard winter.

Still, even if we are in general a slighter species now, we are not, on the whole, meant to look like the models so many of my clients report to be their gold standards. Very few of us will naturally look like Twiggy, Kate Moss, or Naomi Campbell.

Understanding that few of us *should*—and that we all have very different bodies that should look as different as our faces do—is something most of us haven't really learned. And contrary to popular belief, it's not just women struggling with body image. *GQ* makes many grown men expect that everyone with a penis should have a six-pack, and as a result, many men won't take their shirts off when they're mowing the lawn in their own front yard. It's not our fault. In the United States, we've been programmed to think thinner is better.

The Thin Ideal

As a nutritionist, I often hear intimate details about how my clients compare their bodies with others'. They talk about siblings and parents, of course, but more frequently than you might expect, they talk about strangers—the woman in the Nordstrom shoe department, the clerk at the grocery store. At restaurants, we count calories on other people's plates. We are excellent at judging the health of people we don't know. There's a scenario that plays out in my office more often than I'd like to admit. I find it embarrassing. It goes like this: A woman walks in. She's made an appointment to work on "general health" or "low energy," which, from a nutritionist's standpoint, are often euphemisms for "weight loss." She sits on the couch. She looks at me. She bursts out laughing—or crying, one of the two—and drops her head in her hands. "*You?*" she practically wails. "How are *you* supposed to understand?"

Because we have been so over-inoculated with the idea that unnatural thinness is what we're striving for—a concept often termed "the thin ideal"— many folks assume that people just a little thinner than them are healthier (and often smarter, more energetic, or luckier). **That health and size are two different things is a totally foreign concept to most Americans.** It's true; I don't have daily battles with my weight. (I do still have daily battles with food, and I'll get to that later in the chapter.) But the fact that an average person can look at me, someone with an extremely unhealthy history and some still-unhealthy habits, and assume that I'm completely healthy because I fit society's "norm," is plain wrong.

More than once, I've had a mother come in with a teenage daughter who they both believe to be overweight. The mother is tiny. The father is reportedly larger, perhaps a former football or hockey player. She has another daughter who's slim, but the one in my office is built like her dad, and she's clearly tortured by being the bigger girl. She's spent ten years idolizing Disney princesses. Like so many well-meaning moms, this mother wants only the best for her kids. She wants me to help her young girl lose weight because she wants to see her succeed for the rest of her life—she wants her to get a good education and marry someone who makes her happy, and in the mother's mind, this all starts with being thin, even at the age of thirteen.

In my mind, it's much like the tradition of foot binding in China, where for centuries, girls had their feet bound because small feet were believed to encourage a woman's chances of a good marriage. As much as the ideal of a three-inch-long foot now seems ridiculous for anyone looking to spend any part of her life, say, walking, forcing the bigger daughter to adhere to the thin ideal is also sentencing her to a lifetime of pain. With these well-meaning but potentially destructive mothers, my job is much more about changing the *perception* of health than it is about changing health itself. It's about stopping the habit of accepting the thin ideal as it passes from one generation to the next.

The thing is, our desperate yearning for the thin ideal is more extreme than that classic two-daughter family. One study reported that more than half the females surveyed between the ages of eighteen and twenty-five would prefer to be run over by a truck than be fat, presumably because being flattened by a vehicle hurts *less* than the emotional pain of being larger. Two thirds would rather be mean or stupid than fat. I've had multiple mothers bring in their three-year-olds for weight loss. Often, people who find out they need to undergo chemotherapy are relieved at the prospect of finally losing weight. One terminally ill client came to me for weight loss—not because she wanted to live longer, but because she wanted to look thin *in her coffin*. Our culture is that deranged.

What I often teach is twofold: First, I remind people that most models meet the medical criteria for anorexia, that their pictures are digitally edited by professionals who specialize in erasing any perceived defects, and that, eventually, many of them become very sick (and sometimes die) from lack of nutrition. Second, I emphasize that there's a very problematic confusion in America between "healthy" and "thin." Many female soccer players, for example, have natural body mass indexes in the technically obese range, because they have so much muscle mass. Bodies naturally come in a very wide variety, just like heights and skin colors. It's true that overeating and not exercising can lead to poor health. But connecting these unhealthy actions with being overweight is a fallacy. The opposite is also true; the documentary *Fed Up* points out that 40 percent of "thin" people have excess body fat, yet aren't considered unhealthy. Just as there are thin people riddled with depression, poor digestion, and weak immune systems (as I once was), there are overweight people who are happy, strong, and healthy in all measurable aspects. Judging a person's health by their weight is akin to choosing a car based on its paint color.

We each need to accept our own ideal weight. (How's that for easier said than done?) Linda Bacon, author of *Health at Every Size: The Surprising Truth About Your Weight*, has done groundbreaking work that helps our society shift our focus from weight to well-being. She explains that though the personal path we each have to forge independently toward acceptance is very difficult, it's crucial to recognize that we are all born into different bodies. We are not all Disney princesses. We are not all WNBA players. As Bacon argues, I believe finding health requires moving past the thin ideal.

Fattism

Learning to accept our own weight is difficult because our society mistakenly associates being overweight not just with being unhealthy, but also with being weak and lazy. In a powerful TEDxWomen talk, educational consultant Lynne Hurdle-Price talks about the country's *normalization* of looking down on anyone who's overweight. She says it's "the last socially acceptable form of outright discrimination in this country." It's a powerful statement, but it's true. When beautiful women, full of incredible life experience, sit across from me and pour their hearts out about their weight-loss struggles, I often wonder when our society will stop. When woman after woman tells me her husband has offered her some crazy incentive to lose thirty to fifty pounds—a trip to Hawaii, in one case, or $10,000 in another—do you know what I really want to say? I want to say, "Hey, I know how you can lose two hundred pounds in only one day. Dump your husband!" I'm sick of the pressure men are putting on my clients and, more importantly, the pressure these women are putting on themselves. At what point are they allowed to enjoy life and stop worrying about what other people think of them? At what point do my clients get to think that their size is okay? There's this general perception that weight can be completely controlled by willpower, which is totally false. Thin people are not better people. Thin people are not smarter or healthier or more determined people. We work hard to help our clients realize that we want to see them for who they are, not what size they are.

Fattism—the practice of believing that thin people are inherently better than fat people, and that fat people should be actively trying to change who they are because their bodies don't fit the thin ideal—needs to go the way of racism and sexism. Let's kick it out. Let's take a stand by uniting against the culture of oppression that overweight people—women in particular—have endured. Let's cultivate love for the bodies that nurture us and make us individuals, no matter what size, and celebrate our diversity.

A Culture of Shame

We need change on a social level. We live in what I sometimes call a "shame-infested" nutrition culture. Fattism and the thin ideal cause people to feel flawed for simple actions that might otherwise be pleasurable, such as having dessert or skipping a workout in favor of a date with a friend. Brené Brown, the influential author of *Daring Greatly* and an expert on shame and courage, says shame is a powerful and debilitating emotion that's sometimes confused with guilt. (She explains that the classic way to distinguish between the two is that a guilty person believes "I did something wrong" whereas a shame-filled person believes "I am wrong.") Feeling guilty can motivate us to be accountable for our actions, but shame usually has the opposite effect because feeling worthless encourages depression, not action. If we're ashamed of being overweight, for instance, the thought of working out at a health club intensifies the feeling, so we stay home to avoid it. Shame, which we might not even know we're harboring, can surface as anger, isolation, avoidance, and a host of other negative behaviors.

One of my clients, David, reported being so ashamed of his body that every time he went on a beach vacation, he set up an itinerary so detailed that there was no way he'd be able to go to the beach. He organized cultural events, fishing charters, and meals out—anything to avoid actually sitting down and taking his shirt off. Since the vacations ended up being more expensive that way, he felt compelled to work more, which meant he didn't have time to take proper lunch breaks and was constantly running into a bakery next to his work for quick snacks. When the vacation time eventually came, his wife was usually angry that they didn't spend any time on the beach, which made him feel even more humiliated. His entire life was ruled by shame.

Shame undermines our efforts to be healthy, but finding your own ideal weight and health can help push shame out. **Your "ideal weight" is the weight you maintain when you're eating nutritiously and getting**

adequate physical activity. At this weight, you eat well most of the time, you feel good when you move, and you learn to love your body.

The path toward this ideal weight isn't always easy, but it's easy to identify its beginning. It starts with listening to your body.

How to Listen to Your Body

If I were a nutritionist practicing in any other part of the world, I would probably starve from lack of business. I say this because people in most cultures do something Americans have forgotten how to do: they listen to their bodies before, during, and after eating.

In the United States, we stink at listening. We might listen to the easier stuff—when it's time to go to the bathroom or go to bed. But many of us have become so disconnected from our bodies that we don't understand how it feels to be hungry. We think about food in terms of calories consumed instead of what we need. Listening to your body means stopping to tune in to how it is feeling in the moment. Ask yourself: *Am I hungry? Am I full? Am I almost full?* Try thinking about eating the same way you think about crossing a busy street. Before you do it, stop, look, and listen. Ask yourself the same questions you internally file through when you step into a crosswalk: *What's going on? What do you see coming? Can you hear anything different around the corner?* In this way, you can begin cultivating an awareness about your own appetite.

What Does it Mean to be Hungry?

Years of dieting have taught most of my clients that any messages the body sends should be ignored. Most diets are studded with rules, few of which have anything to do with hunger: don't eat meat, eat mostly meat, eat fruit only at a certain time, eat fruit all the time . . . The rules are endless and usually contradictory. The rules make us crazy. They apply someone else's idea of caloric intake to your unique body. Diets condition us to believe that our body lies to us, it cannot be trusted, it will betray us—and worse, that eating isn't actually connected to hunger. But if you listen to your body's true hunger signals, most of the time, you will eat food in appropriate amounts when you need it. You won't eat all the time; a body's wisdom doesn't deceive the way the ego does.

Eating disorder expert and author Jessica Setnick has what she calls the Apple Test: If you are hungry enough to eat an apple, you are actually hungry. Eating when we are hungry implies that we consult our body before feeding it. Ultimately, it necessitates believing that our body knows its nutritional needs and appropriate weight better than we do.

Note that hunger looks different for everyone, and it changes from day to day. On some days, our food choices may seem peculiar to others, but we'll know they're right for us. It takes practice. When it comes to hunger, we usually listen to what other people tell us before we listen to ourselves. Say, for example, that a friend asks you out to dinner. When he asks you what you're hungry for, it may take a concerted effort for you to answer honestly, instead of throwing back the culturally fashionable answer, "Oh, I'm easy. Whatever you'd prefer."

Stop to think about what you actually *feel* like eating. When you do, you've made a conscious effort to listen to your body's wisdom—that internal knowledge that's always there, always ready to tell you what you need. When you're at the restaurant and you order the first thing on the menu that pops out at you (instead of ordering the salad you think you're supposed to eat), you're listing to your body's wisdom. It's the same wisdom our ancestors used to help them determine which foods were safe to eat, when it was time to eat, when it was time to stop eating, and how to prepare foods in new and creative ways. Ten thousand years ago, researchers and authors weren't telling people what and how to eat. People listened to their gut, to that internal and ancestral body wisdom that resides inside the body's second brain. This is your intuition.

Journalist Malcolm Gladwell, in his book *Blink*, talks about how we can fairly accurately describe a person if we briefly look at their car or talk to them for a very short time. The longer we spend with them, however, the less accurate we become because we have a lot of information clouding our vision. This happens with food as well; your first reaction is the most trustworthy. When I started trying to heal myself, I was confused about food because all the books I read and the practitioners I saw flooded me with contradictory information. Nothing worked for me, and so I was left with no option but to sit with myself and try to get in touch with my body. I stopped worrying about the intricate details and started paying attention to my "blink reaction" to foods.

It worked. And it taught me that, when it comes to our bodies, we are our own best experts. Our blink reaction to food is the one we need to learn to trust. More than any doctor, nutritionist, spouse, or coworker, we alone know what we need. Trusting ourselves to know which choices to make when we're hungry is the foundation of reestablishing our relationship with food.

Let's Talk Chocolate

Many women consider chocolate to be their kryptonite, a weakness that surfaces most typically just prior to their menstrual cycle. They blame themselves for having a "fattening" emotional crutch. But we don't crave chocolate because we lack willpower, we crave it because our bodies are smart. Chocolate is high in magnesium, which acts as a natural muscle relaxant and can help ease cramps (plus it tastes good and helps improve our mood). This example can be extrapolated to almost everything we suddenly feel we "need" to eat; we crave certain foods for a reason.

The Difference Between Hunger and Food Cravings

Food cravings are either physiological or emotional or a combination of the two, but either way, they sometimes impede our food intuition. To quiet them, it's helpful to understand the difference between food cravings and hunger, and why we crave foods in the first place. Food cravings demand we eat certain things, while hunger is just the body's signal encouraging us to eat. Cravings aren't "normal." If our body gets and absorbs proper nutrition, we still desire certain foods from time to time, but we don't *crave*. The food no longer dominates us. Instead of making food choices in what become, in effect, emergency situations—when that alien inside steers us off the freeway for a giant bag of potato chips or an ice cream cone because we haven't eaten enough fat that day, for example—we eat what we need to, when we need to. Food cravings are the body's cry for help.

In previous chapters, I've addressed many of the physiological imbalances that result in cravings—not getting enough beneficial bacteria, fat, protein, and calories are four of the major offenders. We may also crave things if our body isn't properly absorbing foods, which means we need to address gut health.

Emotional food cravings, though, are triggered by a feeling, not a biological need. Some of us carry around a host of triggers—an argument with Mom, a tight deadline, anxiety over an upcoming event, or a shameful experience. When we eat or don't eat in response to an emotion, we aren't listening to our body wisdom. We are covering up, drowning out, or burying an emotion that we don't want to feel at the moment. Emotional eating is fairly easy to recognize, especially once we get into the habit of listening to our body.

Of course, human nature plays a part in food cravings too, especially when it comes to sugary foods. Unlike in most cultures, where a three-layer cake might be enjoyed at celebrations or as a special treat, in the United States, sugar-loaded desserts are ubiquitous but have become taboo. So instead of offering us happiness without strings attached, that cake becomes a "forbidden food" that makes us feel deprived and disconnected when we can't have it. We create internal lists of "bad" foods in an effort to curb habits we see as detrimental to our health and weight.

For example, one of my clients chose to walk completely out of her way to avoid even glimpsing a cupcake in a window—because she realized that when she passed the shop, she either felt incredibly sad that she "couldn't" have one and pined for it all day, or she'd walk in, order three with the intention of sharing them, and eat them all. Of course we want that towering cake or the cupcake in the window if we categorize it as "forbidden." It's human nature. But if we're avoiding sugar and not getting enough protein, the result of restriction tends to be total chaos when we finally let ourselves have the forbidden food. The body goes into Last Supper mode, prepares for caloric Armageddon, and as a result, that three-layer cake is gone by morning.

The goal isn't to erase cravings entirely; they're the body's way of communicating. But we want to hear cravings as a low hum rather than blaring heavy metal. We want to make the body less desperate for the things it needs. Healing physically and emotionally is the best way to diminish cravings. In the meantime, we can rely on a few solid strategies for preventing cravings from dictating our diet (see box, right).

The downside to cravings is not so much that we have them but that our reactions to them are detrimental. Our first reaction is to blame ourselves. We spiral into shame and self-hatred. Really, the body is sending us a message: it's simply out of balance, and it's trying to tell us so.

More times than not, I see that balancing clients' general physiology greatly diminishes their cravings. People are usually amazed, because they have always labeled themselves in certain ways—they lack willpower, so they just can't have cheese or ice cream in the house, for example. I tell them that if they're craving cheese and ice cream, that's a strong sign that they are not getting enough fat in their diet throughout the day. Making a delicious adjustment can change the way you eat and how you feel about yourself.

Take a Stand

When I work with clients on trusting body wisdom, some of them have to let go of powerfully engrained beliefs around what they should and should not eat. Trusting body wisdom takes courage and time; it's not easy, and it doesn't happen instantaneously. It requires that we take the "shoulds" and

Tips for Controlling Emotional Eating

Eat with other people.
Clients of mine who are immigrants often say that they never had a problem with food until they moved to the United States. Back home, people ate together and prepared meals together. Mealtime was very social. Eating in isolation after a bad day is a setup to overeat. Creating social meal times can help immensely.

Practice preventative eating.
If we have had a tough day and come home from work starving, we can easily make it pull-up-a-chair-to-the-fridge time. Why wouldn't we? We are hungry and upset, and we start eating randomly. Some chips, crackers, yogurt . . . and then all of a sudden we are not hungry for dinner so we continue to snack all evening, ultimately consuming more food than we would have if we had a balanced meal and a conscious snack. Practice preventative eating by planning mini meals. Try tapas (Spanish appetizers)—for example, marcona almonds, olives, cheese, dried fruit, and salami, which can be kept in your office and don't require preparation—not something light like a piece of fruit, which is not substantial enough. If you work a nine-to-five shift, I recommend eating around three or four o'clock. It can make a huge difference in the evening.

Listen to some upbeat, happy music.
If you're prone to overeating or bingeing, music can instantly change your mood and diminish the appeal of overeating. This is a good strategy to use in the car on the way home, when you might be tempted to hit the drive-through, and during dinner preparations, as you're deciding what to eat.

"should nots" out of our vocabulary. But once clients start trusting themselves to eat what they need, when they need it, a few things happen, both personally and politically.

First, you might go through a temporary phase where all you want are foods that have previously been off-limits. If you've avoided fat for years and finally reintroduce it to your diet, you may go through a time when it's all your body wants. When I returned home after spending a month in China, where people don't consume a lot of dairy, the first thing I did was eat an entire stick of butter—I plopped it onto a plate and ate the whole thing. Luckily, I didn't freak out. I trusted my body to know there was something (most likely fat) I had been missing while abroad and that I needed it.

Although I eat some butter almost daily, I haven't had the same all-out craving for it like I did that one time. Today, I trust that butter will be there for me if I need it again, but I don't fear it. Trust that the foods you want to eat when you start giving yourself permission to eat whatever resonates with you are usually temporary. For some people, it lasts a day; for others, it goes on for weeks. For ten days straight you might eat bananas dipped in peanut butter for breakfast, lunch, dinner, and snacks. Please know this will not last forever. Eventually your body will move toward something different.

Next, expect that your thoughts about food and eating, as well as your eating behavior, will become more peaceful. Instead of devouring an entire container of ice cream, you might be surprised to be satisfied with a bowl. When you stop prohibiting your body from eating what it wants, you'll stop eating to satisfy some unmet physiological or emotional need.

Also, don't be surprised if you begin eating tastier foods, but smaller quantities of them. Listening to the body usually teaches my clients that the low-fat or low-calorie foods they'd been accustomed to eating simply don't taste as good as the full-fat or regular versions. In most cases, they enjoy "real" versions of their favorite foods and find them much more satisfying. They order what they want at restaurants, which can be scary at first. They make what they actually desire for dinner. Typically, this renewed focus on enjoyment leads to being more present during the process of eating— before, during, and after—which means you'll hear your body when it says it's full.

Any kind of change, whether positive or negative, brings loss. Learning to listen to your body is no exception. We gain something, in the form of health, but lose something too. Many clients, before committing to trusting the body's innate wisdom, spend an inordinate amount of time thinking about what they're going to eat next, feeling guilty about eating, and searching the cupboards or the market for the next snack. Like a recovering drug addict who needs to fill the time he previously spent buying drugs, taking drugs, and thinking about drugs, you might grieve the empty space that you once filled by obsessing about food and beating yourself up about eating.

Developing Intuition

Even if you're starting from scratch, developing body wisdom is possible. Here are some exercises, inspired in part by Evelyn Tribole, a pioneer of the intuitive eating movement, that you can use to try to find that wise place inside you—the one you can depend on day in and day out for all your decisions, not just those related to food:

- At restaurants, ***order the first thing on the menu*** that pops out at you, even if it doesn't make sense.
- For three days out of every week, ***eat exactly what you want for your afternoon snack***, from popcorn to cheese to potato chips to truffles.
- For three days out of every week, stop and ***ask yourself what it is you really want for dinner***, and do what your body tells you, even if it means a peanut butter and jelly sandwich.
- ***Include a dessert a week*** that you really want. Stop, breathe, and tune in to assess what it is. Get exactly what you want, even if it doesn't make sense. If it's a double-baked almond croissant from a bakery all the way across town, have exactly that. If you can't get it that day, tell yourself you'll have it the next time you pick up your dry cleaning nearby. Following through establishes trust between you and your body.
- ***Slow down.*** Eat with chopsticks or your non-dominant hand, if it helps. If you're loading up your fork so the fork is waiting in front of your face, full of food, for the entire time you're chewing, you're eating too fast. Practice breathing between bites and putting your utensils down occasionally. Eating slowly allows your brain to tell you when you're satisfied and gives you time to ask yourself how much you need.

continued

- If you eat and then are hungry two hours later, before you usually have your snack, eat again. Listen to your body and *eat when you're hungry*. This will also establish trust between you and your body; it will learn that you will listen.
- If you go to the county fair with your kids and you really want a corn dog, have it. *Enjoy random food run-ins*, knowing that events like the fair are occasional.
- *Eat gratefully* when you're not in charge. Say you go to your family's house for Thanksgiving, and they don't cook much from scratch. Enjoy every bite of the cranberry sauce that's still imprinted with the ridges from the can, the boxed stuffing, and the marshmallows on the sweet potatoes. How often does someone prepare a meal for you? The stress hormones you release panicking about high-fructose corn syrup and hydrogenated oils are probably more damaging than the food itself is, and Thanksgiving comes once a year.

The process of letting go can be terrifying, but it's also liberating. Freeing up the time we previously spent worrying about what we ate leads to more important changes in how we function every day. We think more clearly. We have more time to spend succeeding at whatever we do. When we feel better, we have more self-esteem, which allows us to reach beyond the societal habit of defining health by what the media tells us. Trusting your body allows you to stop worrying as much about how others judge you and ultimately take a stand against the young/thin ideal our patriarchal society ties to female success. It helps you remember who you really are.

What Your Eating Habits Say About You

There is a huge psychological component to eating. Over the course of my career, I've noticed patterns that link the way people eat to their underlying emotional state. Do any of these ring true for you? You may be a combination of two or three, or perhaps you were once one, and now you identify with another.

The Worker Bee

Everything happens in a rush. You're typically totally stressed out and busy, and people you know admire how well you balance a family, work, and social life. Although you can usually justify eating quickly, or at your desk or in your car, you're often using your schedule to avoid some buried emotions. You may feel like you're always running away. Worker bee foods: crunchy, salty things and one-pot meals (often unbalanced) that are easy to prepare.

The Sitter

You're the world's caretaker. When you eat, you tend to be totally present. You almost always sit down for meals. You often eat very slowly, focusing on your meal and savoring each bite. People tell you you're very grounded. Ultimately, you're good at listening to others and to your body. Sitter foods: warm, long-cooked foods, like soups and stews.

The Roller-Coaster Rider

You're on a never-ending guilt trip. You're very good at following the rules, but often out of touch with your true wants and needs, both at work and at home. Socially, you let others make all the choices. Inside, though, you feel totally out of control. It's the same with food. You follow dieting rules out of shame about your weight or appearance, and are often very rigid and self-judgmental. Eventually, you binge or overeat, then feel extremely guilty, which perpetuates a cycle of loss of control. Roller-coaster rider foods: baked goods, ice cream, and chocolate.

The Snake

Like so many snakes, you tend to eat all at once, often in huge amounts once your hunger has reached its climax. Your thinking in general tends to be very black and white. Your friends commend you for being bold and believing so strongly in yourself and often, for achieving so much. You tend to prioritize everything over your health and your needs, though, and flexibility isn't your strength. You frequently skip meals, "forgetting" to eat, thinking that you'll take better care of yourself once some stressful event is over, but the process of forgetting and then starting to starve makes you eat huge quantities when you finally eat. Snake foods: big meals, like a double cheeseburger with fries.

The Rule Follower

You listen well and follow directions, both in life and in the kitchen, but you apply other people's rules to your own body even when they may not be right for you. You're confused about what you eat and what you want, and you just wish someone would tell you what to do. You're constantly hungry, because you spend so much time picking apart what you should or shouldn't be eating that you've forgotten how to enjoy food. Rule-follower foods: classic diet foods, such as raw vegetables, low-fat dairy, and lean meats.

The Planner

In your life, everything requires a plan. When you lie in bed at night, you plan the next day's foods with the same precision as you plan big events. You follow a regimented exercise routine that you always adhere to, even when you're sick. During the day, your dominant thoughts are about food—what you'll eat when, how eating one thing should affect what you eat next, and what you'll eat tomorrow. Social situations are challenging because you lose control over your own food choices; you often skip parties at the last minute because you know any deviation from your plan will require you to beat yourself up mentally for days after. Planner foods: low-calorie snacks; boneless, skinless chicken breasts; steamed broccoli; brown rice.

The Satisfied Customer

In social circles, you're often the spontaneous, flexible one, the person everyone thinks is fun to be around. You trust your instincts and your intuition. At restaurants, you order the first thing on the menu that pops out at you.

Your food choices don't always make sense to other people; what you eat changes with the seasons and with how you're feeling. Satisfied customer foods vary wildly.

Learning to Incorporate Forbidden Foods

It's worth repeating that it may take time for your body to recognize that it doesn't need some of the foods you're used to eating. Once it does, it's usually important to reintroduce "forbidden" foods to your diet; it's a valuable step toward healing your relationship with food. When diet-minded clients have trouble letting go of "forbidden" foods, I recommend they make dates with the things they love.

After changing their protein intake, I get many e-mails from clients reporting that they can suddenly keep ice cream in their freezer for the first time, when for months or years, they've avoided it because they could never have just a little. Ice cream is a classic excess food; it's something people open and eat right out of the container, often until they're scraping the bottom, without really thinking about what they're consuming. They eat totally mindlessly. The goal is to move away from ice-cream gorging and back toward what could be termed the Ice Cream Date. Although this tactic isn't limited to ice cream—it works for anything you crave that you feel you probably should eat a little less of, or that you know you sometimes eat without really enjoying—it's a useful example of how to approach "forbidden" foods.

First, establish with extreme clarity what it is that you want. If it's ice cream, is it deep, dark chocolate or just regular chocolate? Or do you want that new coffee kind you heard the neighborhood ice-cream shop is making? Choosing the flavor your body tells you it really wants is a way to establish trust between you and your body. Next, make a plan. It may be easier at first to eat it in a shop or in an individual serving size because it's a safe, controlled setting. (If you're at home, be kind to yourself; buy a small container instead of the gallon-size tub.) Finally, enjoy a real serving, in a real bowl, and sit down to eat it. Really *enjoy* it. Moan, if you need to.

When you're finished with your date, think about whether the ice cream satisfied you. Recognize how your relationship has changed. Are you sated? Are you full? When you put the bowl in the sink, wash away any shame or guilt you might associate with that food as best you can. Those negative feelings do nothing to help you. Instead, embrace the satisfaction associated with the food, and think about the possibility of changing your relationship with it. You can make an appointment with the freezer for the same time the next week, if it helps, or decide what flavor you'll get on the following date. Ideally, over time, your body will stop giving you uncontrollable urges to eat and the food will become an enjoyable, occasional part of your diet.

Moving On

That our hunger and cravings may have more to do with our physiology and hard-wired emotions about weight, instead of just about willpower, is a huge change in the way most of us think. It's hard to listen to our own body's wisdom instead of what the media says. It's really, really hard. Remember that while it sounds easy on paper, the process of moving on—moving from a place where we freak out about everything involving food to the place where we just enjoy eating—is something that will take time. (If it wasn't hard, my clients wouldn't come back just to be reminded, over and over again, that eating isn't something they should be ashamed of.) If you drift away from accepting your body's wisdom and its history, gently encourage yourself to try again. I know it takes time because I've helped thousands of clients walk this slow, sustainable path to self-acceptance, and I've walked it myself.

Today, I still have daily battles with my body. Even though I live a "normal" lifestyle now, I hoard food. It's in the cupboards, for sure. But it's also in the coat closet, the car, my backpack and office, the basement freezer, the bedroom and bathroom, in pots and pans, and inside the salad spinner. I'm terrified of being without food. When I traveled across South America, I carried salt, pepper, and a bag of rice with me for two months, even though I had no way of cooking. Because I spent so long without enough of it, food gives me security.

Although it functions for me in a much different way than it does for many people, I think relying on food for security is quite common. Know that while you may do your best to move away from using food as a crutch, your history will always be part of who you are. The goal is embracing a healthy, successful future, but it doesn't mean you have to erase the past.

Moving forward, keep focusing on the Living in the Gray Guideline (see page 53). Try to eat what your body tells you to eat most of the time. Try to forget the thin ideal most of the time. And, most of the time, try to push past any shame you associate with eating and listen to your instinct. But the other little slivers of time that remain, let yourself be whoever you are, eat whatever you end up eating, and move on. For me, that often means forgetting to eat, because I'm so well trained to accept being hungry. I work on making a concerted effort to listen to my body and being okay with how my past has made me who I am today.

Most importantly, moving forward means trusting yourself. If the media tells you red wine is good for a healthy heart but you think red wine makes you sleep poorly, your body's wisdom beats the research. If I tell you that you need a certain amount of protein but you come to realize you need more or less, follow your intuition. You're the expert. Don't let anyone— not the magazine covers, not nutrition labels, not me—tell you differently.

What You Might Be

Lao-tzu, author of the *Tao Te Ching*, says that when you let go of what you are, you become what you might be. He was a philosopher, but I'd like to think he'd have made an excellent practitioner at Passionate Nutrition, because his words echo what we believe. The foundation for the acceptance we hope every client can find—the altering of the deeply engrained belief that thinner is better and that body size alone determines intelligence, beauty, or diligence—is letting go of past beliefs. When we trust our bodies to know what is best, they trust us back. Over the years, we've found that once clients reach a stage of happy self-acceptance, they often lose weight simply because they've found peace. Shedding the fear and sadness that has plagued them for so long is a huge physiological relief. When, after the course of months or years, they are finally able to let go of the labels they've plastered onto their bodies, they notice a complete paradigm shift. They're no longer obsessed with calories. They forget they have a scale. Acceptance leads to a freedom most clients have never known.

....

THE PRESCRIPTION

- If it applies to you, think about admitting that you may be addicted to feeling bad about yourself and your body.
- Recognize that history, media, and culture play a huge role in how we feel about our bodies.
- Practice listening to your body to determine what you want to eat and how much your body needs.
- Experiment with enjoying eating.
- Eventually, think about reintroducing "forbidden" foods to your life.
- Work toward letting go of past shame and guilt and moving toward a more accepting, trusting, loving relationship with your body.

Chapter 9

THREE INGREDIENTS
for NATURAL BEAUTY

If you and I, every time we pass a mirror,
downgrade on how we look or complain about our
looks . . . we remember that a girl is watching us
and that's what she's learning.

—Gloria Steinem

There's a huge state fair in Washington every summer, with corn dogs, big rides, aging rock stars, and miles of well-groomed animals—the whole shebang. I stepped up to the ticket booth one September, at age thirty-nine, and the cashier paused. "Student or adult ticket?" she asked. My friend's jaw dropped open. The student ticket cutoff was eighteen.

I look good, but that hasn't always been the case. As a kid, acne ruled my life. I always felt like everyone was staring at my face; I wore hoods to cast shadows over my cheeks. So many times, I debated making a headfirst dive into a patch of asphalt on purpose, thinking that any resulting scar would be better than what I saw in the mirror every day. I connected my skin problems to my self-worth. Acne made me feel dirty. I just wanted to look like everyone else, but I didn't have the money to buy the products I thought would change my life.

Image forms a huge part of our identities—not just for women, but for men as well. When our skin or hair fails us, we feel debilitated, because part of that identity has been altered or stripped away. We stress constantly about our faces, our hair, any rash or spot. We all remember embarrassing teenage years to a certain degree. When people don't like something about their appearance, they feel helpless. But those of us who have bounced from specialist to specialist know that our modern culture's approach to cultivating smooth skin, glossy hair, and strong nails doesn't always work. What Western medicine gives us is more of a patch that works temporarily but doesn't solve the underlying problem.

A Flawed Approach

Our culture's approach is broken in more ways than one. More than *how* to make ourselves more beautiful, I struggle with *why* we think we need to. I realize that I'm partly in the business of beauty, yet I hate and reject that the world expects us—especially women—to look a certain way. I hesitate to even include this chapter: Why should we be pretty? But whether we like it or not, beauty opens doors. We "dress up" for meetings, dates, and occasions. Defining beauty by how we (or our significant others, siblings, or bosses) think we look rather than by our happiness and how healthy we feel is a huge cultural flaw. With my clients, I make it a point to differentiate between beauty as defined by mass media's airbrushed, male-defined, oversexualized, stick-thin models and natural beauty, which is what we all have when we are well fed and well cared for (and have enough calories to think clearly and powerfully). Beauty is feeling good *inside*, not looking good *outside*.

Notice, in the pages that follow, that I will never ask you to change who you are. I will never help someone with lighter skin achieve darker skin, or vice versa. I never recommend hair coloring, straightening, or extensions. I'll never tell a teenager she'll "grow out of" her weight, skin, or hair; teaching young girls that something about their body needs to change inherently sets them up for a lifetime of eating disorders and poor self-esteem. Telling women they're imperfect because they don't look like a magazine cover cuts away at their power and potential. And while, in many cases, the onus is on men for creating false feminine ideals, it's up to women to learn— and crucially, to teach—that beauty comes from the inside. At Passionate Nutrition, a firm that employs forty powerful women, part of our mission is to empower our clients and change cultural habits surrounding beauty.

But while I grapple with our society's (largely male-dominated) definition of beauty (Thin body! Clear face! Long hair!), it's also my job to help people feel good. When I help a client deal with a lifelong eczema or acne problem, it's about comfort, not about what her boss or neighbor sees or says. Beauty tips are a dime a dozen; my goal is to help women feel good so they can be personally and politically powerful, not so they can look like America's Next Top Model. The kind of beauty I advocate is empowering, not enslaving. It means we spend less time and money trying to look good because we feel good in our bodies from the moment we wake up in the morning—before we look in the mirror, before we ask our partners to tell us how we look, before we walk into the world to find out who likes our new hair color. And it starts, not surprisingly, with eating well.

I See Your Face

I've learned to find beauty through food. By the time I was eighteen, without the vitamins and minerals a body needs, I was a wreck; I was living off sugar and I didn't drink water. I worked at Club Fantasy at this point, so I had to look good; I relied on makeup to hide my real skin. In the two decades since, a system reboot has turned me into the woman on the cover of this book.

Food leaves its fingerprints all over our bodies. We are what we absorb, yet despite decades of being told to "eat healthy" in order to be well inside, few of us connect what we put in our mouths and on our bodies with what we see in the mirror. At the same time, that reflection rules us.

Sometimes, I just wish my clients could see what I see. In China, there's an ancient practice of face reading that I began learning when I was traveling there. According to practitioners, a person's face is said to reveal traits about their personality, nobility, wealth, and luck, just to mention a few. It's a lifelong pursuit—one I certainly don't claim to have mastered in my short study—but that experience taught me how much I can learn about nutrition just by looking at someone's face. When clients walk in, I don't usually notice that they have heavy earlobes, for example, which in physiognomy, as the face-reading practice is called, indicates a generous and considerate person. I do notice the finer details. If the earlobe has a deep diagonal crease, the person usually has lots of underlying inflammation. Drawn, wrinkled skin points to a lifelong low-fat diet. Dark circles under the eyes can indicate an iron deficiency. Dry skin with eczema usually needs more essential fatty acids. Red, cloudy whites of the eyes tell me the body's liver is being overworked and that the client needs more fruits and vegetables. Most of my clients have grown used to masking these problems instead of solving them. Usually, the mask comes in two forms: makeup and medication.

Cosmetics are a $55 billion industry. In the United States, we spent $3.6 billion on makeup alone—and that was in 2011, during a recession. We work hard to make the money we spend on products that cover up the way we look, but we don't typically consider that the skin underneath all that concealer is made up of what we eat and drink. We have the power to change it simply by changing our eating habits. Eating for the way we look—and how we feel inside, top to bottom—is an easy, tasty way to overhaul the body. It's often much less expensive than makeup and certainly cheaper than many "magic" treatments (think Botox and chemical peels).

Likewise, Americans spend huge amounts of time and money seeking medications to cure what I, as a nutritionist, see as obvious nutritional deficiencies. Many of my clients will spend a Saturday afternoon diligently shopping for and preparing organic whole foods, then head to the mall on Sunday to fill their bags with facial products packed with dangerous chemicals. I teach people how to run fewer errands; most of the products on Sunday's list do the same things foods can do, only food makes permanent changes, often for less money—and, if you're eating whole foods, without the chemicals. Everything from chapped lips to flaky nose creases can be improved with food. I don't think my clients need more pills—they just need proper nutrition and to absorb their food better. They need to start at the cellular level, so when I address beauty, I start with addressing cellular health. And healthy cells start with eating enough fat.

What I See

Below is a list of some of the most common symptoms I see at Passionate Nutrition, along with what I often suspect to be the problem.

- **Acne (face and back):** Too much refined sugar; deficiencies in vitamin A, zinc, and essential fatty acids (EFAs)
- **Bags under eyes:** Dehydration
- **Dark circles under eyes:** Iron deficiency, allergies, or poor kidney function
- **Dandruff:** Too much refined sugar; deficiencies of EFAs, B vitamins, or selenium
- **Diagonal earlobe crease:** Inflammation highly associated with cardiovascular disease
- **Dilated capillaries on cheeks and nose:** Too much alcohol, poor digestion
- **Dry hair:** Hypothyroidism; deficiencies of EFAs or iodine
- **Dry skin:** Hypothyroidism; deficiencies in vitamins A and E, biotin, and EFAs
- **Easy bruising:** Deficiencies in vitamins C, K, and bioflavonoids

continued

- **Hangnails or cuticle inflammation:** Deficiencies in zinc, vitamin C, folate, and protein
- **Petechiae (small pinpoint hemorrhages found all over the body):** Vitamin C deficiency
- **Poor nail growth:** Mineral deficiency, poor digestion
- **Premature graying:** B vitamin deficiency
- **Rosacea (redness of the forehead and cheeks, with pimples):** Poor digestion, possible carbohydrate sensitivity
- **Nails with horizontal or vertical ridges:** B vitamin deficiency, poor digestion
- **Skin tags:** Warning sign of type 2 diabetes
- **Varicose veins:** Deficiencies in bioflavonoids, vitamin E, magnesium, and fiber
- **Vertical line between eyebrows, with swollen edges:** Liver congestion
- **White spots on nails:** Too much refined sugar, zinc deficiency, possible gluten intolerance

Beauty Secret #1: Eat Fat

For most of us, the word "fat" induces fear. But from a scientific perspective, fat is a molecule that plays many more roles than what we see on our plates—and few of them are visible to the naked eye. Let's talk about health on a cellular level.

Every single cell inside the body relies on fat for flexibility and nutrient transport. The cell walls have to be strong enough to keep what's inside in and infectious intruders out, but flexible enough to permit smooth passage of nutrients, fluids, and waste as well. Fats give us the right balance of rigidity and flexibility in each and every cell, which helps us achieve the optimum level of health. With fat, our bodies look and feel better because our cells work better.

By contrast, long-term low-fat diets leave cells too inflexible. Without fat, the cells have trouble both accepting nutrients and getting rid of toxins.

For our skin, this translates to wrinkles and poor nutrient balance, which can cause many of the complaints we've all had at one time or another—dry or flaky skin, acne, rosacea, eczema, spotting, and hair loss, to start. And for each external change we notice, there are likely three or four internal problems we never see. Inside, fats support the proper function of the immune and hormonal systems, and also facilitate vitamin transport and absorption. (Note: The brain is 65 percent fat too.) Many of the ailments we suffer from every day can be traced back to a simple lack of healthy fats.

But while we often focus on how much fat we take in, we should really look more closely at what *kinds* of fats we consume. Cold-pressed and unrefined oils such as extra-virgin olive oil are good plant-based sources, as are coconut oils and fatty plant foods such as coconut products, nuts, and avocados. However, the optimum balance of the rigidity and flexibility required for good nutrient transport depends on getting a mix of fats. Unsaturated fats, which we get from plants, make our cell walls more flexible, while saturated fats, which we get from animals, make them more rigid. We need both.

Essential fatty acids (EFAs) are short-chain fatty acids our bodies require to function; they're called "essential" because our body can't make them. They transport vitamins A, E, K, and D throughout the body and help regulate mood and inflammation. On the skin front, EFAs do a lot to control inflammation and regulate moisture content; getting enough can combat inflammatory skin issues like eczema and psoriasis. The bad news is that we can't make all the fatty acids we need ourselves, and there are quite a few of them. We need omega-3s such as eicosapentaenoic acid (EPA) and docosahexaenoic acid (DHA) to survive, yet we don't have any sort of biological bank that keeps them at the ready. The good news: we can eat EPA and DHA in grass-fed beef and cold-water fish.

But while we recognize that we need fatty acids, most of us don't realize it matters where we get them. Alpha-linolenic acid (ALA), for example, is found in plant sources such as flaxseeds and nuts. While we can convert ALA to EPA and DHA inside the body, it's much more difficult for the body to perform those conversions when it starts with plant matter. When it comes to EFAs, eating fish can be as much as ten times as beneficial as eating plants. So while many vegetarians and vegans may be consuming EFAs at a rapid rate, their bodies may not actually be getting the benefits they need.

Typically, if we listen to our taste buds, we have an inherent instinct that tells us which fats work best for what we're eating, so over the course of a few days, we eat the right combination of fats to benefit our bodies and skin. If someone plops a baked potato in front of you, for example, chances are you'll want butter or sour cream (both saturated fats), not olive oil (which is unsaturated). But if you're going to make a salad dressing, few of us use melted butter; we use olive oil. We all know that. Still, decades of fearing saturated fats has made it difficult to accept that they're required for healthy, supple skin, strong bones, and a healthy immune system.

Saturated Fats Are Good For You

Saturated fat is so named because of how each carbon atom in the fat molecule is "saturated" with hydrogen; it means the fat is solid at room temperature. There has long been a fearmongering connection between heart disease and saturated fat intake, but based on the prevalence of fat in other cultures' diets and their commensurate low rates of heart disease, the connection doesn't hold water. Prior to the 1920s, heart disease caused less than 10 percent of deaths in America. By the 1950s, the rate had risen closer to 30 percent. As a result, America turned its attention toward lowering fat and cholesterol intake, and, as I discussed on page 113, accepted the lipid hypothesis as a general rule. Today, we blame heart disease for 35 percent of deaths.

Ironically, in 1965, a study reported in the *British Medical Journal* followed patients who'd already had one heart attack; they were asked to ingest plain corn or olive oil to see if that might decrease cholesterol and thereby boost longevity. Two years later, those who used corn oil had far lower cholesterol than the others, but only 52 percent were still alive, compared to 57 percent of those who used olive oil and 75 percent of the control group, which consumed (saturated) animal fats. On a cultural scale, it was a matter of traction. That the lipid hypothesis, which was based on a very small sample of data, became more popular than the 1965 study was basically a fluke.

Saturated fat plays a crucial role in our body systems. Sally Fallon, president of the Weston A. Price Foundation, founder of the Real Milk campaign, and well-known nutritionist, explains the role saturated fat plays in the body: It makes up almost half of each cell's membrane and protects the liver from the toxic effects of drugs and alcohol. It plays a vital role in bone health; at least half our fat intake should be saturated if the body is to absorb calcium effectively. It has antimicrobial properties that protect us from pathogens. And it often comes paired with cholesterol, facilitating hormone function and lipid digestion.

While the generally accepted norm used to be that cholesterol is a precursor for heart disease, scientists have now realized that cholesterol is so important that asking people to limit intake may in fact be harming them. The American Heart Association has now recognized that the one thing people with heart disease all have in common isn't cholesterol, but inflammation. Today, heart disease research reveals that it's better managed by reducing inflammation, decreasing the amount of dietary trans fats, and managing blood pressure. There's also evidence that decreasing the amount of polyunsaturated vegetable oils we eat—oils like corn, canola, and soybean—may decrease the threat of cardiovascular disease.

On the face front, eating fats from a variety of sources—in foods like olives, avocados, coconut, fatty fish, beef, butter, and other dairy products—translates to better absorption of vitamins A, D, E, and K, which play big roles in controlling acne and dry skin. To quote Julia Child, if you're afraid of butter, use cream.

The Bad Fat

Although saturated fat has been emancipated from its former negative labels in most scientific circles, there is still one type of fat that is best avoided: trans fat. Now illegal in some states (but still lurking in some packaged foods), trans fats are made by bubbling hydrogen gas through refined oil, which saturates the oil with the gas, making it resistant to oxidation. In other words, it turns fat into a preservative. Trans fats can lead to heart disease, cancer, diabetes, decreased immunity, and obesity. Avoid any product that has the words "hydrogenated" or "partially hydrogenated" in the ingredients list.

Beauty Secret #2: Drink Water

Another crucial part of eating, which is easy to overlook when we're so focused on food, is drinking. Staying hydrated is crucial to good health; think about how sad an underwatered plant looks. Water makes up 78 percent of the human body, so it's important to get enough of it. Every day, clients walk in totally dehydrated, with bags under their eyes and often with complaints about dry skin, fatigue, and constipation. Most of these problems improve when we simply drink enough water.

I explain dehydrated cells to my clients with what many anatomy and physiology professors call the "balloon theory": When a balloon is full of air or water, it has more surface area than when it's all shriveled up. That's the way our cells work too. When they are plumped full with water, they have a much larger surface area and so are able to absorb nutrients and rid the body of waste products much more easily and effectively. Remember: healthy eating is not just about how many nutrients we eat, but also about how many nutrients our cells are able to absorb.

Short-term dehydration causes inconvenience, but over the long term, it can be quite harmful. Bags under the eyes turn into creases, wrinkles, and dead skin. Constant constipation can lead to bacterial imbalances and intestinal inflammation—even intestinal permeability (which means small particles of proteins and partially digested foods get absorbed through the stomach's lining and passed into the bloodstream before they're ready to be used there). Dehydration can also put too much pressure on the kidneys, which in turn tell the body to conserve water, leading to bloating and fluid retention. In general, water keeps us looking and feeling younger for longer.

Water also eliminates toxins. To understand how this works, imagine doing dishes. Think about how rinsing out a sponge with water cleans the sponge: clear water goes in, we squeeze, and murky water comes out. Without that water, all the stuff that was in the sponge just stays in, and the sponge gets smelly, moldy, and funky. (Eventually, we usually throw it away.) Think of your body as the sponge. Clean your sponge!

I recommend clients carry a 32-ounce water bottle with them most of the time, and make it their goal to fill it and drink the contents twice each day, primarily between meals. It is ideal to drink water that is room temperature or warm; cold water can be shocking to the system because the body is required to work hard to warm it up. Ditto for chlorinated water; the fewer chemicals in our water, the better. However, the priority is getting water; temperature is a secondary consideration.

On the flip side, drinking too much water during or after meals can dilute the concentration of acids and enzymes needed for proper digestion. Think of your stomach as a fire that is constantly ready to burn up the food you eat; drinking water puts out the fire. I recommend people avoid drinking a lot of liquid twenty to thirty minutes before *and* after meals. (If you need to take supplements or any other pills with food, try to use as little water as possible to swallow them.) There are, of course, exceptions, and they're often liquids some cultures have been consuming with meals for centuries. Tea, wine, or other digestion-promoting beverages that are fermented or have digestion-enhancing spices are okay.

If you feel like you need to drink a lot of liquid with meals, it could be a sign that you're not chewing well enough. Focus on chewing slowly and consciously, which I know is easier said than done. (Try some of the techniques listed on page 161.)

Water Fight

I hear from clients that it's always a fight to drink enough water, so I spend a lot of time focusing on how to make it easier. Hydrating doesn't mean you always have to drink plain water, which is a relief for people who find it, well, boring. I make it more tempting for the kids in my house by keeping a big pitcher of water with something colorful (such as berries) inside, so that when they open the refrigerator, that's their first option. If you have trouble drinking enough, try adding the following to make it more interesting:

- Handful of smashed blueberries
- Five or six cucumber slices
- Juice of a lemon or lime
- Splash of apple cider vinegar
- Sprigs of mint, thyme, or rosemary
- Sliced oranges (room temperature or frozen)
- Handful of melon cubes
- Herbal tea bags
- Big pinch of salt

Remember that, as with most things, drinking water isn't all or nothing. Do what you need to get the water in, even if it means adding a little juice.

Beauty Secret #3: Incorporate Seaweed into Your Diet

According to dermatological studies, zinc plays multiple roles in protecting the skin: It enhances wound healing, protects against harmful UV rays, and controls oil production. An imbalance of zinc (or especially, a deficiency, which most of us have) can lead to acne, scarring, and photosensitivity. Zinc is key to skin health. Yet doctors lead suffering teens and adults alike to dangerous oral medications, often without even asking them what they eat. And it's likely that, as an adult, while you're obsessing in front of the mirror about this red spot or that wrinkle or *akk! another zit!*, still no one has recommended you get a little more zinc into your diet. No one has probably ever told you that eating more seaweed could save you a lot of time spent in front of that mirror.

It's true, and it's that simple. Seaweed has vast benefits for skin because it's mineral-rich. Both eaten and applied topically, seaweed solves a wide range of persistent skin problems, from acne and dryness to redness and rosacea. Besides zinc, it contains selenium, which offers our skin natural protection from the sun and increases its elasticity, and silica, which strengthens the body's connective tissues. Seaweed also contains low levels of copper, which acts as a general anti-inflammatory. (You may have seen people with arthritis wearing copper bracelets for the same reason.)

If you're prone to acne, for example, you may need beta-carotene, which is found in arame, nori, and kombu—an easy trio to get in a single dinner at a local sushi restaurant. If you have dark circles under your eyes, you may need more iron, available in arame, dulse, nori, and wakame. Iodine, the frequent cause of dry hair, is something all seaweed contains. In general, any seaweed variety you find, fresh or dried, will make you look and feel better, period.

Day-to-Day Beauty Basics

As I discussed in Chapter 3, food that's not really food can make us sick. Similarly, we should take care of our skin using products that are as natural and chemical-free as possible; what we put on our skin gets absorbed directly into our body. First and foremost, this means focusing on eating foods that can beautify us from the inside out. (Eat more fat, and plenty of it. There, I said it again.) Because many common cosmetic products contain harmful toxins—everything from hair straighteners to nail polishes to deodorants can be dangerous—I try to keep my own use of these to a minimum. I recommend you do your best to avoid products that contain butylated hydroxyanisole (BHA), boric acid, lead, parabens, coal tar, formaldehyde, petroleum distillates, phthalates, and all artificial fragrances. It may sound like I'm recommending you skip performing radical science experiments on your face, but look into the ingredients in the products you use daily; you may be surprised by what's inside. Just like you do with food, avoid using anything on your skin, hair, or teeth that you can't identify.

On a daily basis, though, I agree we need some basics. We need to care for our teeth and skin. Most of us like being clean. (I shower twice a week, because I think, in general, we are an overclean society. I reserve soap for my underarms and butt, so as not to disturb my skin's natural bacterial balance.) I'm not asking you to go without deodorant, but if you're open to it, I'd strongly recommend trying inexpensive, natural alternatives to what you currently use. There are many good products available at natural foods stores, but my favorites come from the kitchen. I use baking soda on my underarms. I put coconut oil on dry skin and calloused heels, and if I notice dandruff, I rub my scalp with olive oil. Following are the products and rituals I use to keep my skin clean and clear, my hair shiny and strong, and my teeth healthy.

A Beauty Regimen from the Kitchen

When I make my beauty products—it seems strange to call them that, but that's exactly what they are—I don't measure, because it takes too much time. My mornings need to be simple. Learn to estimate; these combinations are very forgiving. You'll notice they have very few ingredients, which means they're easy to incorporate into a daily routine (not to mention cost-effective compared to most peoples' bottled beauty supplies).

The Morning Ritual:
Simple Baking Soda Face Wash *or* Exfoliating Oatmeal Face Scrub + Apple Cider Vinegar Toner + coconut oil for moisturizer + Baking Soda Deodorant

The Nightly Ritual:
Oil Face Wash

The Twice Weekly Ritual:
Baking Soda Shampoo + Apple Cider Vinegar Conditioner

The Weekly Ritual:
Seaweed Softening Bath + Simple Seaweed Mask + occasional Coconut
Hair Conditioner

The Mouth Ritual:
Baking Soda Toothpaste + Coconut Oil Mouth Detoxifier + Natural
Whitener

Recipes

Simple Baking Soda Face Wash

Blend ½ teaspoon baking soda in the palm of your hand with enough water
to make a paste. Spread the mixture over your skin as you would a facial
wash, then rinse.

Exfoliating Oatmeal Face Scrub

In the palm of your hand or a small bowl, blend together 1 tablespoon
rolled oats, ¼ teaspoon sea salt, and enough water to make a paste. Spread
the mixture over your skin as you would a facial scrub, then rinse.

Apple Cider Vinegar Toner

In a glass jar with a lid, combine 1 part apple cider vinegar with 2 parts
water. After washing your face, apply the toner with a cotton ball, then
apply a moisturizer, such as coconut oil.

Baking Soda Deodorant

For each armpit, blend about ¼ teaspoon baking soda with enough water
to make a paste, and use your fingertips to rub it in. (Do not rinse.) I keep
an open bowl of baking soda near my sink. After I wash my face, I simply

dip my wet fingertips into the soda, and it always seems to be just the right amount.

Oil Face Wash

It sounds strange, but yes, using oil to clean your skin works amazingly well, even if you wear makeup. In a small bottle, blend together one part castor oil and three parts extra-virgin olive oil. Rub about a teaspoon of it into your face in small circles for about a minute. Wet a washcloth with hot water. Place the cloth over your face and let it steam your skin until the washcloth cools to room temperature. Gently dab the oil off your face with the washcloth. (You can use extra oil to remove any makeup that hasn't already come off.) All done! Do not wash, use toner, or add lotion afterward. If my skin feels especially dry, I just sleep with the oil on and skip the washcloth part.

Baking Soda Shampoo

In the shower, spread 2 tablespoons baking soda into the roots of your hair, using your fingertips to rub it into your scalp. Rinse with warm water.

Apple Cider Vinegar Conditioner

After shampooing, drizzle 2 tablespoons Apple Cider Vinegar Toner (see page 183) over your hair, rub in, then rinse away.

Seaweed Softening Bath

As your bath water runs, add to it 1 tablespoon coconut oil, 1 cup whole milk, and ½ cup dried or powdered seaweed (any kind). Ideally, add the ingredients to a very hot bath, and sit until the water is no longer hot, up to an hour or longer. When you get out, pat yourself gently dry instead of scrubbing, so the coconut oil stays on your body. (You can add ginger, cinnamon, oats, lemon, or lavender too, depending on what scents appeal to you.) If you don't have time for a full bath, try the same recipe for a foot soak.

Simple Seaweed Mask

In a food processor or coffee grinder, grind 2 tablespoons dried seaweed (any kind) until powdered, or buy it powdered. If you have makeup on, first wash it off. Mix a tablespoon of the powder in the palm of your hand with enough water to form a paste. Spread the paste on your face and let it sit for thirty minutes, then wash your face and moisturize with coconut oil.

Coconut Hair Conditioner

When I feel like my hair is becoming brittle, dry, or frizzy, I give it a coconut hair-conditioning treatment. Use a tablespoon of coconut oil to coat wet, clean hair, especially at the ends. (The amount you'll need will depend on how much hair you have; you can take just a dab at a time, letting it melt in one palm and then applying it bit by bit, repeating until all the hair is covered.) Wrap your hair in a rag or a sheet of plastic wrap (or you can use a plastic bag) and sleep with the coconut oil in overnight before rinsing in the morning. (Depending on the look you're going for, you may need to wash your hair. If you're going for a slicked-back style the coconut oil will be fine.)

Baking Soda Toothpaste

I use that same bowl of baking soda by the sink to brush my teeth. Morning and night, I wet my toothbrush, then press the bristles into the baking soda and brush as with toothpaste. If I notice stains on my teeth, I dip a cotton swab into the baking soda and use it to scrub the stains.

Coconut Oil Mouth Detoxifier

In traditional Ayurvedic medicine, the process of swishing with coconut (or sesame) oil is called oil pulling; it's long been known as a detoxifier. After brushing, put 2 teaspoons of solid coconut oil into your mouth. It will feel strange as it melts, but it will indeed melt after about thirty seconds. When it's turned to liquid, begin swishing, as you would with mouthwash. Continue swishing as you go about your morning duties; the oil will pull saliva into your mouth, so you'll have more to swish with. Swish for twenty minutes total, if possible, before spitting out everything in your mouth. Swish with water and spit again. I try to do this daily.

Natural Whitener

Once every week or two, I use hydrogen peroxide as a natural tooth whitener. Put about 2 teaspoons of hydrogen peroxide into your mouth and swish. It gets all foamy and doesn't taste particularly good, but leave it in your mouth until you can't stand it anymore, for about ten minutes, if possible. I keep inexpensive hydrogen peroxide (the same ingredient in most expensive teeth whiteners) in the shower, so that I can whiten while I bathe.

In general, I recommend the Environmental Working Group's guide to skin care products; see EWG.org for more information.

Bone Broth for Skin, Hair, and Nails

Because it contains gelatin, collagen, and elastin, bone broth is an excellent source of nutrients for skin, hair, and nails. It's sometimes called "beauty broth" for good reason! (See page 241 for a recipe.)

Keep It Simple

I once had a conversation with a sorority house mother who couldn't get over how her girls were ruining all her cast-iron pans. "They refuse to cook with fat!" she complained. Over time, the pans got dry and completely scraped up; the gals totally abused them. As grown-ups, most of us know food will stick to the pan if we don't grease it in some way first. If you care about your skin, hair, and nails—and most of us do—it may be easier to think of your body as that cast-iron pan. All day long, add plenty of fat, then let your body do the cooking.

As with eating, live in the gray when you care for your skin. If you're at a hotel for the weekend, you will survive without coconut oil. Seaweed may be harder to come by if you're at a work conference in Paris. (Also, lucky you.) The rest of the time, get plenty of fat, water, and seaweed, and be prepared to see a new you.

....

THE PRESCRIPTION

- If you're unhappy with the clarity and glow of your skin, experiment with adding more fat to your diet.
- Carry a water bottle and try to drink at least 64 ounces of water each day.
- Incorporate small amounts of seaweed into your diet regularly.
- Play with using natural beauty products instead of any that might contain toxins.
- Define beauty on your own terms.

Chapter 10

GOOD FOOD, GOOD SEX

Do you want to meet the love of your life?
Look in the mirror.

—Byron Katie

For years, I thought I was broken. Deep down, I really believed that I was utterly and irreversibly broken by my past. That a generous, abundant, enjoyable vitality—let alone sex—would never be part of my life. That having sex was just a role for me to play when I needed to service a man or make some money.

Actually, no. I was worse than broken. I believed I was sexually cursed—by my childhood sexual abuse, my mother's ironically puritanical values, and my job as a sex worker. Those things, plus the fact that I could never have an orgasm. Sex wasn't something to be savored, enjoyed, or appreciated; from a too-young age, it was my job, as was taking out the trash and occasionally mowing the lawn.

Even though they helped, it wasn't the hours of reading and therapy that led to my eventual sexual epiphany. It was simpler than that: I learned to love. I learned to trust the person I was with, a woman, and learned to listen to myself. Before, sex had been a performance, and that performance always had to be good. When I was with a man, I felt like I had to prove my worth. My sex-addicted father had instilled in my sister and I the twisted idea that women existed only to be sexualized and that no one over a size 8 (yes, there was a cutoff!) was worth a man's time. My income—my very livelihood—had at times depended on it.

When I was alone, I cleaned my body with a washcloth (because Grandma always told me it was wrong to touch myself, even in the shower) and created very strict rules governing my relationships: No clothes off until the ninth date. No sex until three months had passed. What my own body felt physically or emotionally had nothing to do with what happened when I undressed. My body was simply a tool. Being with a woman changed every-thing, because I didn't feel any pressure to give a movie-quality performance. Suzanna, my first real love, showed me the patience and kindness and inti-macy sex requires. She taught me to relax, breathe, and feel. Eventually, at age twenty-eight—a full sixteen years after I lost my virginity—I had my first orgasm. I thought it was a fluke. Even though it kept happening, for years I was terrified the magic might go away. It wasn't until I learned to love myself—and forgive myself and my family for every bit of my past—that I accepted I could heal, and that enjoying sex was a critical, curative, *healthy* part of being a woman.

My history is unique, but I know I'm not alone. Most of us are sexually impaired in some way. Many of us still haven't achieved orgasm and have adopted the habit of just getting sex over with, regardless of how much we actually like it. We ignore it, then we avoid it, then we rush it.

It's no wonder. We're all busy people. For most women, the day steam-rolls us before we realize it, and as a result, we have nothing left to give our-selves or our partners by the time we crawl between the sheets. You get up each morning, and if you're lucky, you have a minute or two (but no more) to yourself. You get the kids up, make breakfast for the family, get your partner out the door, fix yourself up, organize your thoughts for a client meeting, race through work, and grab something to cook for dinner on the way home.

You pull duty as the unpaid fourth-grade math tutor, cook dinner, fold laundry, break up a fight over who gets to feed the fish, put the kids to bed, and finally collapse into bed. Your partner, whom you truly love, turns to you and says, "It's Wednesday, baby," which is code for "I want sex." You do it because you think it's your duty, but there's really nothing in it for you. All day, you give and give and give, and at this particular moment, you have just one more thing to give before you get what you want: sleep. You make it as quick and easy as you can, regardless of whether you actually orgasm. It's the sexual version of fast food. And actual sexual gratification is often low on your partner's priority list because it's just as low on yours; why would someone want to please you if you don't seem to care about pleasing yourself? Somehow, you two never get around to talking about it.

In this last chapter, I'm going to talk about sex—specifically, why we don't talk about it, what that does to our experience with it, and how we can change our relationship with sex by changing our relationship with food. Though I'm a nutritionist, not a sex therapist, over the years, I've found that an important part of the healing that comes out of my food counseling reveals itself in the bedroom.

The Great Taboo Topic

Sex is one of our culture's biggest taboos—besides maybe poop, I can't think of anything people feel less comfortable talking about, especially in mixed company. (Chances are you felt reasonably comfortable buying this book, but wouldn't dare buy a sex-therapy book in public.) Yet we see sexual images every day. Sex is used to sell everything from cola to cream cheese to cleaning supplies. Our society commodifies the female body because we've grown used to connecting images of beauty with our own success—*that gorgeous woman eats Greek yogurt for breakfast, so I'll be happy and sexy like her if I buy Greek yogurt*—yet the unspoken rule is that women are supposed to be sexual without expressing their unique sexuality. When it comes to our pleasure, there's often no real conversation between female friends beyond half-drunk whispers on ladies' night, and usually even less of a rapport between us and our partners. Women are expected to keep their bedtime routine to themselves during the day, but transform into sex kittens for their partners at night. We live that Usher song "Yeah!" with its lyric, "We want a lady in the street but a freak in the bed."

But it's hard to be a sex kitten when we're never taught to learn how to make sex enjoyable. Telling women, either directly or through cultural channels such as movies and television, that they have to give sex but don't necessarily have to enjoy it is a crushing American cultural habit. Fathers give sons the sex talk, but it rarely, if ever, includes paying attention to how the girl in question feels. Mothers give their daughters cautions, not tips on how to feel good with a partner. (My own mother never had an orgasm.) How are we supposed to enjoy sex if we never learn how to talk about it and never learn that feeling good about our bodies is part of it?

Sex and Shame

If you look back through history, you'll see we've made a huge departure from previous traditions when it comes to the culture of sexuality. Most ancient cultures operated by a matriarchal line that prized feminine libido (and in fact, sometimes feared it). As Nancy Tuana, a Pennsylvania State University professor and author of several books on women and sexuality, points out, ancient Greeks thought women to have many times the desire for sex that men had. In her article "Coming to Understand: Orgasm and the Epistemology of Ignorance," she quotes Apollodorus as saying that for every ten "parts of love's pleasures," a woman takes nine and leaves one for a man.

In ancient Hindu texts, it's clear that orgasm is thought to balance the chakras, and that an imbalance in the lower (sexual organ) chakras is thought to be the root cause of most diseases. (Susun Weed, author of *Down There*, recommends seven orgasms a week to promote female organ health.) Chinese medicine thinks of sex as being energizing and nourishing for women. Ancient yogic texts taught that the only way to reach enlightenment, to know God, was through sex. It wasn't until the nineteenth century, according to Tuana, that the image of women as extremely sexual beings shifted—and, not surprisingly, when that happened, a newfound ignorance about orgasms in general demoted women in society.

Even then, I'd argue that this shift perhaps only permeated the Western world. When I was studying at an ashram in India with a group of nutritionists and naturopaths, we had whole classes that addressed healing frigidity in women, which was classified as an actual illness. (At the time, I recognized I was the woman they described, and felt completely broken and dysfunctional.) But somewhere along the way, Western society devalued women's pleasure as a means of controlling it and controlling women themselves. Victorians covered table legs to avoid any possible turn-ons, and mothers started teaching their daughters that they needed to rein in their sexuality and cover their bodies. We began passing shame down from generation to generation. Posturing as asexual became the norm. Although we've recovered somewhat, there's still a culture of shame surrounding our bodies and our sex drive, which hurts the power of women in general.

Today in the United States, sex is such a taboo topic that it's lost its intrinsic human value. Women here are as ashamed of their actions or thoughts as they are of their bodies, when in many countries, both are still a highly prized part of life. (Latinas, for example, are known for being "sexy" because they embrace a more voluptuous feminine ideal. When I was traveling in South America, women didn't seem ashamed of their curves or their sexual desires. The same goes for other places I've traveled, including Italy, South Africa, Central and South America, and Fiji.) Our shame forces us to hide who we are sexually, which in turn injures our self-esteem and teaches us to edit our emotions. Sex is a biological urge. On some level, we all want it, and we all need it. But the inherent shame engrained in sex in this country—shame about our body parts, what we did as young adults, even shame about sexual orientation—translates to an entire society built on silencing how women feel about sex.

In modern history, we've accepted a role as the silent partner. When women *want* in the most sexual way, they're often considered dirty, rather than powerful; we have perceived limits to where we can go in the bedroom, because typically, we let men lead. When women aren't happy with their sex life, there's no outlet. We're just stuck, which impacts our perception of personal power, and, ultimately, our happiness.

Think about the last time you got together with a group of girls for drinks. (If you're a man, my apologies. Consider much of this chapter a learning experience.) Chances are you'd have no problem plopping down with a big sigh and complaining about feeling fat or discussing your latest diet strategies or griping about your children. You'd probably get a chorus of compassion. But if you sit down and say, "I'm feeling really lonely and I'm bad at masturbating" or "It's really been a long time since I had an orgasm," you'd hear a pin drop.

That we're this uncomfortable talking about sex says two things: first, that complaining about our bodies is the only socially acceptable way of complaining about underlying sadness and anger, and second, that we're missing an opportunity for growth and sexual healing by avoiding discussions with the very women we consider our closest friends. When we let go of that shame surrounding sex and begin discussing sex itself, we discover that our stories are often the same. We de-isolate ourselves. We bond as a gender, which enables us to reclaim, in part, the sexual power we had in the past.

What we often find, when we start talking about sex, is that it's more of a spiritual practice than a simple act. Now, after a lot of work addressing my beliefs about what my role was with a man (see How We Find Self-Love on page 202) and learning to trust that what I feel is important, I am no longer ashamed of my body or my history. I now see sex completely differently; I take time to prioritize and enjoy it because I've realized it's the crux of my emotional balance. I couldn't have made these strides—and evolved away from the shame I once felt surrounding all things sexual—if I hadn't purposefully and specifically decided to change my role from giver to taker also and to begin *enjoying* sex.

Let's Talk About Sex: Three Questions

The next time you feel an emotional rush about sex—it could be anger, sadness, or extreme happiness—remember it and think about sharing it with a woman you trust. Talk about sex. Although it might be funny, it's not quite as effective if we just say, "So, tried any new positions in the sack lately?" Being vulnerable helps others feel comfortable opening up. Here are three questions that can help bring up sex in conversation in a gentle way that encourages group participation. Ultimately, the goal is to be as comfortable talking about sex as we are chatting about our kids or gardens.

1. The other night, my partner accused me of liking sleep more than sex. What do you think? What if I do? Is that a bad thing?
2. I've been feeling sort of powerless about a lot of things in my life. What do you think makes women powerful?
3. Do you think good sex is essential for happiness?

Sex Is Good for You

In the same way that we're all built to think certain foods taste good, every woman is biologically built to experience pleasure. Like food, we *require* it for nourishment. Just like every animal—there is hard evidence that we're not the only mammals to experience orgasm, and that masturbation and homosexuality are quite common across species—we need sex to satisfy physiological needs.

Some of the benefits of sex are obvious. According to many studies, the simple act of touching—a hug, for example—can lower the heart rate and calm the nervous system, thereby easing tension. (I think part of what feels so healing about seeing good friends isn't just talking things through; we also feel the physical effects of the hug that often preempts and concludes conversations.) Sex also takes energy, and we all know exercise is good for the heart.

Not surprisingly, sex plays an important role in our hormonal pathways too. Cortisol, for example, which is referred to as "the stress hormone" because the body releases it during times of stress, tells the body when to divert resources away from "low-priority" functions such as immunity, bone growth, collagen production, and fertility, and toward higher priorities, which, historically, meant more "traditional" stressors, like surviving when hunting a man-eating beast. As a hormone, cortisol is quite useful when we need to survive, but from a health standpoint, it can be detrimental if the body produces too much of it. Unfortunately, many of our stressful cultural habits also increase cortisol—think caffeine, sleep deprivation, and even commuting.

In females, because oxytocin (which is often called the "bliss hormone") suppresses the cortisol response, one of the keys to controlling stress is improving oxytocin production. Women release oxytocin upon orgasm, and in this case, more is better; frequent orgasmic sex decreases stress even more. But most of us can't flip the switch that changes us from stressed to turned-on quite so easily.

The research suggests that the acts we engage in surrounding sex—talking, cuddling, or connecting on some intellectual and emotional level that makes us feel less alone—are chemically helpful. For both men and women, talking and sharing stimulates oxytocin production and reduces stress. One study in *Biological Psychiatry* showed that "social support," defined in the study as time spent with the subjects' best friends, had an anxiolytic (anxiety-reducing) effect on the subjects after they were exposed to a stressor. So while sex itself—and specifically, orgasm—can help decrease stress, the precursors to sex may also be good for achieving high levels of oxytocin (and could get you in the sack in the first place).

Sexual Healing

I've established that sex is healthy for us. That said, instead of thinking of our bodies as shameful or undeserving of anything but total satisfaction, we should think of them as assets. *Being* sexual requires *feeling* sexual. We have, residing quite conveniently inside of us, the power to make ourselves feel ridiculously good and release the negative effects stress has on the body in one fell swoop. When we hate our bodies or feel anxious when people look at us, we block our ability to feel sexual. When we understand our bodies and learn to ask for what we want and need, we unleash that powerful tool and learn how to use it to our own advantage.

For those who find orgasm embarrassing, unnecessary, or meant strictly for a man's pleasure, sexual healing often comes in the form of liberation from the cultural misconception that we have sex strictly for conception. Many women can identify with that feeling of "going wild" that resonates within the moment of orgasm. Daniel Vitalis, whom I once heard speak at a conference that focused on sex, advocates a "rewilding" of humankind that replaces the idea of any shame or guilt associated with sex with the acceptance that humans, like many animals, can have sex for fun. (It's pleasurable. It lowers stress. We should do more of it.) This concept—that having sex can be a selfish, self-serving event—helped emancipate me from my abusive past and learn to enjoy it.

Of course, some of us just don't *want* to have sex. It's become boring, exhausting, or embarrassing, or some combination of a whole host of negative things. It may not be that we harbor unnecessary shame surrounding our bodies or the act of sex itself, but simply that our partners haven't helped us become aroused. In that case, sexual healing means figuring out how to get turned on in the first place.

This is why sex experts like Dr. Tammy Nelson, author of *Getting the Sex You Want*, says that if you want to have sex with a woman on Saturday, you have to start on Wednesday. Sex hormones and stress hormones are very interrelated. They play many different roles in balancing each other, but stress trumps sex every time. Think of it this way: If you're being chased by a tiger, you don't want to feel aroused—you want to run. It's always a delicate balance, but by stimulating oxytocin before sex, you can get your body away from its natural stress response.

It's not that the sex hormones have no fighting chance, it's just that we have to be deliberate in flipping our physiology into that mode. Ergo, women who have help handling stress in their day-to-day lives, in the form of the talking or cuddling I mentioned before, often have lower cortisol (stress hormone) levels, and hence higher libidos. (Pay attention, men: this means listening and helping around the house are actually proven chemical pathways to sex.) It's no accident that I had my first orgasm with a woman who listened to me every day and provided me with consistent emotional support. She knew what I needed. With her I could relax, which meant I could lift the iron gates I'd always posted in front of sex. (Ultimately, she helped me learn what I'd need to be happy with the man who is now my husband.)

But some of us don't want sex because we've gotten really good at telling ourselves we're just not worth it because of how we look or something we've done. I don't always talk to my clients about sex, but when I do, it typically revolves around connecting how we love with how we eat. There's a lot more common ground between sex and food than you may suspect.

Sex and Food

When I address the intersection between sex and food with clients, I start by talking about stress. Of course we're stressed in our daily lives. It's hard to avoid, especially when things like work and kids come into play. But sadly, for many of us, the simple, required act of eating, something we do multiple times every day, often causes more stress than the body can handle. We have to say no, over and over. In our diet-focused world, it irritates me that so much of our day focuses on what we can't do—no carbs, no fat, no snack after dinner, no cupcakes, no this, no that, no *freedom*. No enjoyment. And more often than not, the rigidity we place on our diets translates to inflexibility and negativity in the bedroom. (This is where my career walks into your bedroom.)

Imagine what happens when you go to a holiday party, alone or with a partner. Do you eat whatever's passed around? Do you ask what food people have prepared or participate in its preparation? Or do you politely decline anything you're not sure about? If you're the type to dive into the experience and typically enjoy social engagements, chances are you feel more comfortable with your body and with yourself, and are similarly more comfortable in the bedroom. If you find it scary not having full control over what you eat or you don't like eating in front of people, you may harbor negative feelings about your body, which typically translate to poor self-esteem and unsatisfying sexual experiences.

Now expand the dinner party example to the rest of your life. Think about how you live. Do you rush through everything? Do you have set routines that you adhere to every day, no matter what? Do you have rules about everything from what you eat and don't eat to what coat you wear for a certain outdoor temperature? That's stressful. Eating under stressful conditions also makes us release cortisol, which diverts the body's attention away from arousal. Keep in mind that, as Marc David, author of *The Slow Down Diet*, says, how we eat is how we live. How we eat is also how we love. The woman who controls her every bite at the party is probably going to go home angry, guilty, and stressed, and not be in the mood for sex, while the one who ate what the host prepared and had a good time is probably going to be a little more lively back at home because she can love herself even if she eats a few more cookies than she planned. She knows how to let enjoyment take over.

Next, I talk about forgiveness. The common denominator between loving sex and loving food is the forgiveness that allows us to let go of our past. When we learn to forgive ourselves for our mistakes and whatever flaws we may perceive in our bodies, we can learn to first accept and then eventually our bodies. Similarly, when we forgive ourselves for those same things with respect to food—our pasts and our mistakes and whatever flaws we may perceive—we learn to love food, rather than fear or hate it (both of which stress us out from a hormonal perspective). The woman who controls her intake at the party is punishing herself for her perceived flaws; the woman who eats dessert is embracing the moment and has helped create a relaxed, fun atmosphere.

I thought I could never have the kind of sex that actually made me feel good. Similarly, for a long, long time, I believed that nothing I ate could make me feel good either. I associated both sex and eating with pain, shame, guilt, and embarrassment. That I made strides toward enjoyment in both arenas simultaneously is no accident; I learned to take the stress out of both sex and eating by forgiving myself for things I'd done "wrong." When I learned that food could make me feel good, it became simpler than that—after years of being a prisoner inside my own body, I was allowing myself to feel good, period. When I learned I could feel good, I could expand that feeling beyond eating to sex.

Having bad experiences surrounding food is not that different from how women, especially young women, react to a sad or unsatisfying sexual history. With sex, if there's physical pain, they focus on the pain, and the related fear rules their subsequent experiences. If there's heartbreak, they focus on the heartbreak, and rule out any future relationships. We all have these things—past shame about masturbation, awkward first sexual encounters, and the like. Similarly, with food, the pain and heartbreak surrounding past failed (usually diet-related) experiences and how we feel about our bodies stays with us from year to year and prevents us from enjoying food in the future (which, in turn, often prevents us from feeling worthy of enjoying sex). In both cases, with food and with sex, moving on allows us to feel intimacy and enjoyment, which in turn begets more intimacy and enjoyment. But that switch—learning to approach ourselves with love, instead of with shame—begins by addressing the past.

Practicing Forgiveness

Forgiveness is a prerequisite for good sex. Most of us—if not all of us—have issues from our past that creep into our brains now and then and make this seemingly simple concept close to impossible. But how are we supposed to expect others to love our pasts, our foibles, our weaknesses, our bellies, our butts, or our thighs if we can't love them ourselves? The path toward a healthy sex life requires approaching these issues head on.

Start literally. The next time you look in the mirror, practice paying attention to what kinds of emotions cross your mind. Are you sad, angry, or ashamed? Do you see a person, or facts about that person that you like or dislike? Are there things you hide from others that you know you alone can see in that reflection? Do you love what you see? Or do you usually avoid looking in the mirror altogether?

If you feel an abundant, warming love for yourself almost every time you look in the mirror, kudos. (You're probably eating enough fat!) But if, like most of us, you struggle with loving yourself during the day, chances are you don't feel sexy in bed at night, and you don't practice love when you eat. Look for a way to learn to be sexy and healthy from the inside out by forgiving yourself for your supposed imperfections.

Start by identifying just one thing that you think you've done wrong. Maybe you've spent too much time in the sun, and your face has suffered, or perhaps you've been using ice cream to soothe the pain about a recent breakup. Maybe you have a genetic disease, arthritis that causes you pain you're ashamed of, or embarrassing digestive stress. Start with *one* thing. Look in that mirror and forgive yourself. *I forgive you for choosing to marry a man who ended up hurting you.* Whatever it is, say it right out loud. *I forgive you for working too much over the last decade.* It doesn't matter how silly it sounds. *I forgive you for becoming addicted to Snickers and Cherry Coke.* It could be complicated or extremely simple. *I forgive you for fucking up.*

Over time, you'll find that forgiveness has the power to allow us to feel comfortable with ourselves, which translates to better sex. When you love yourself, you tap into a deep well of potential enjoyment that is most readily accessible when you also practice self-love.

How We Find Self-Love

In America, few of us even know how to identify self-love. We talk about body image, meaning how we perceive our bodies, but typically, good body image translates to acceptance or satisfaction, not love. True self-love—a term coined in 1956 in *The Art of Loving* by psychologist Erich Fromm—is defined as loving yourself even when you're honest about your strengths and weaknesses. Most psychologists agree it's necessary to find self-love before someone else can love you.

"Every woman is beautiful in her own particular way," says Eve Ensler, author of *The Vagina Monologues* and influential feminist and activist. Ensler tells a now famous story about a conversation she had with an African woman outside Nairobi. Citing her self-consciousness about her curvy stomach, Ensler describes how the African woman elaborates on how she loves each part of her body and why. Ensler is shocked because in America, we don't cultivate the same kind of love. We don't know how to love our bodies; instead, we cultivate a culture of comparison. If our stomachs and thighs and hips are bigger than our neighbors', we consider them better people. We blame ourselves for not measuring up and consequently feel ashamed of our body parts, so we hide them. The African woman seems confused by this. She points to a tree and asks Ensler whether she thinks the tree is pretty. Then she asks if it's still pretty considering it doesn't look just like the tree next to it.

The point, well made, is that both trees are beautiful, but that their beauty doesn't depend on what they think of each other. We are all our own individual trees. As the African woman says to Ensler, *You've got to love your tree*. No one says it better.

Of course, it's not quite that easy. We all have this tree, this body, that like most trees, has probably been through a lot. When most of us look in the mirror, we see only the negatives, the marks of past storms: saggy boobs, crow's feet, too-curvy hips, and imperfect skin. Self-love means learning to love the whole package, perceived flaws and all.

My path to self-love was complicated, as so many are. My issues revolved mostly around sex, and were more emotional than physical. For years, I did not trust men. I loved and partnered with women, and deeply enjoyed the freedom being with a woman gave me, but wondered whether I should again consider dating men. I went to therapist after therapist to work on my approach to relationships, and one day, one therapist recommended I witness The Work of Byron Katie, an expert in the field of self-love. (I wish Katie's book *Loving What Is* were required reading for all women.) In The Work, which is what Katie calls her simple but powerful method of inquiry, Katie asks her clients to write down the thoughts that have been causing them stress. Once people question these thoughts with the four questions of The Work—"Is it true? Can you absolutely know that it's true? How do you react, what happens, when you believe that thought? Who would you be without the thought?"—their whole outlook on life changes, and thoughts that used to cause fear, anger, or depression lose their power. People return to their original, joyous nature. What is left when the mind can see clearly is more than acceptance of ourselves and our situations: we become lovers of what is.

I first encountered The Work at the nine-day School for The Work with Katie in California. At the School, Katie does a writing exercise on shame, in which participants are encouraged to jot down their most nagging thoughts. We wrote and wrote, and at the end, I read aloud my story about being a sex worker at Club Fantasy, head down, and explained how my history made me a terrible person. I relived the humiliation and discomfort I felt knowing I'd chosen to be paid for sex as a consensual adult. Only afterward, instead of avoiding me as I'd expected, the group rallied around me. At a silent lunch afterward, I intentionally sat at a corner table facing a wall. Slowly, one by one, the entire table filled up. There were no words, but they were there, sitting with me to heal me and tell me I'd made the right choices for myself at the time. It was one of the most pivotal moments in my life.

To share my shame with a room full of people—and have them support me instead of turning away from me like I expected—changed everything about my self-perception. Soon after, I ran to my room and cried. The other participants had found it in their hearts to accept me, but I still hadn't found it within myself. After that day, though, the shame eventually faded away, like ice melting, slowly but dependably. I also left with a newfound discovery that I might not actually be a lesbian; I'd just avoided men and felt safer with women. I became open to the idea of dating men, and in the long run, to the idea that I could enjoy sex on a much deeper level.

Katie's Work taught me that I didn't need to associate my shame about my former life as a sex worker with an inability to be pleased by men. In fact, she taught me to embrace my past, and to use it as a tool to live happily and abundantly in the present. I am grateful to Byron Katie every day for teaching me the skill of self-love.

For me, the path to that love was neither short nor easy, but following it was a decisive part of my happiness today. I learned that for me, sex is a spiritual practice. I can judge my emotional state by my sexual state; if I'm too busy, I don't prioritize sex or I rush it. Giving myself permission to enjoy sex slowly means I'm prioritizing my own needs over the needs of others—something most women find very difficult and something I'd been conditioned to do. Often, when I have a very satisfying sexual experience, one where I put aside all my thoughts about my body, my past, my job, and my chores and focus just on allowing myself to feel good, I feel like I'm experiencing something that benefits womankind on a more global level. If I can put aside my own history, forgive myself, and learn to really love myself, it seems any woman could find fulfillment.

Byron Katie's website, TheWork.com, is an excellent starting point, but talking with friends, relatives, and therapists can be helpful in finding self-love too. Many of us know, deep down, that we need to digest problematic past emotions. But for most of us, we blame our bodies instead of addressing the problems themselves. *If I could just lose fifty pounds, I'd be more self-confident*, we think. Or, *If I can control what I eat, I'll have a more perfect figure*. But the time for finding self-love is not later, when you weigh less or feel better or finally get to go on that dream vacation. It's now.

How to Eat for Better Love

Happily, on the nutrition front, there are things we can do that encourage a new path toward loving our food, which, in my experience, translates directly to how we love ourselves and our partners in the bedroom.

First, learning to eat in a more exciting way can add charge to the boudoir. Just as having sex the same way every time can become boring, so can eating the same foods day after day. When clients come to me with a gray pallor and report a lack of sex drive, I often suggest adding more spice to their diet. Chili peppers, for example, cause the same pattern of sweat and excitement that arousal does, but even milder spices—cinnamon, cloves, and ginger, for example—can increase blood flow in a similar way. In *Psychology Today*, Michael Castleman describes how novelty, the simple act of trying new things, can trigger dopamine release. Just as testing a new position in bed with our partners can increase sexual arousal, becoming more daring with what we eat often translates to more excitement and exploration at home.

You should also eat abundantly. We need food. Because our bodies are hardwired to need and crave calories, restriction requires an enormous amount of energy and self-control. This not only takes away from the energy we might use for sex, but it also tends to bleed out into all aspects of our lives. If we're inflexible about which foods we eat and when, or if we establish rules governing what we're required to do in order to "deserve" certain foods, we become restrictive in all aspects of our lives. If eating liberally scares you, start by practicing with habitual noneating tasks: Leave through a different door to take out the trash. Drive a different way to work. Wear different shoes with a previously planned outfit. Slowly, you may be able to increase your flexibility with food, which translates to more fun in the sack. Eat with the same sense of abundance you'd like to bring to your bedroom.

Did You Know?

In 1894, Dr. John Harvey Kellogg, the man behind Kellogg's cereal, created Corn Flakes to curb the "urges" thought to be created by a breakfast that contained meat, sugar, and other tasty flavors. The blandness was said to squash sexual desire.

Next, though I've said it before, eat enough cholesterol and fat. Our culture has been inundated with the idea that cholesterol is bad for us, when it's actually crucial to the majority of our body's processes, including the manufacture of sex hormones. Cholesterol helps the body use serotonin, which keeps us happy. Without enough cholesterol, we experience mood swings and sadness—not exactly things we associate with coital bliss. In a study on 300 adult Swedish women, those with the lowest cholesterol reported the highest rates of depression. Cholesterol promotes brain cell health and growth too, and regulates the production of estrogen, progesterone, and testosterone. As Dr. Ruth Westheimer famously says, the most important sex organ is the one between your ears. So if you're not getting enough cholesterol to feed your brain, your chances of being both unhappy and unhealthy rise. Cholesterol promotes happiness, and happiness promotes sex drive. It's that simple.

Cholesterol is usually paired with fat, an equally important partner in hormone production. Healthy fat consumption is now linked to decreased rates of Alzheimer's and coronary heart disease, but we are so conditioned to fear fat and prostrate ourselves before the "thin ideal" I discussed in

Chapter 8 that we forget health doesn't have to look like the cover of *Shape* magazine. The models society perceives as those with "perfect bodies" are, in reality, too thin to actually produce sufficient sex hormones. When women are healthy, female hormones produce fat-deposit patterns that typically result in curvy hips, thighs, and buttocks; women who don't have enough fat for their particular body type often struggle with sex drive.

Add Love to Your Plate

Adding love to your plate doesn't mean every meal has to be your favorite, but it does mean you should work on enjoying almost everything you eat. Frequently, this starts with slowing down (or even just sitting down), because it's difficult to appreciate the creaminess of a good yogurt or the sweetness of a strawberry when we're shoveling food in next to the television or at a stoplight in the car.

Think about textures. Think about flavors. Think about what the food is doing for you, the same way you might pause to think about whether something your partner does in the bedroom is working for you. Really *love* the food, and ask yourself whether it's loving you back. (It sounds hokey, I know, but try it. When you eat a meal, ask yourself whether the food you're eating is giving you something you need.) Treating food as something that nourishes, rather than something to be afraid of, ashamed of, or governed by, is good practice for using sex as nourishment too. When we learn to eat food that nourishes us, we get better at choosing people with whom we can share healthy, loving relationships.

The New Healthy Plate

Health requires love every bit as much as it does any vitamin on the shelf at your pharmacy (or in the food at your farmers' market). Forming healthy relationships is the foundation of our society. When we learn to interact in a safe, positive way with our food and with each other, we change our lives. When lots of us do it, we change our culture and empower women, instead of suppressing them. That's why I've included a sex chapter in my nutrition guide. Sex and the love that comes with it is part of good health.

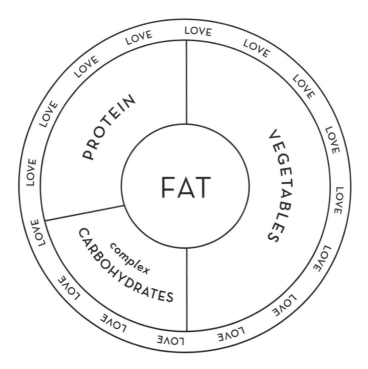

The next time you sit down, think about how you eat. If you're following all ten chapters in this book, you'll likely predict that about half your plate should be vegetables and that you should also have some protein and a good hunk of healthy fat mixed into your meal in whatever form you like best. There might be fermented foods and miracle foods sprinkled in there on most days too. But sitting along the edge of your plate, participating in every bite you eat, should be love—love for your food, which nourishes you, and love for your body, because you are your best asset. Only when we include this love in our meals can we become the best versions of ourselves.

....

THE PRESCRIPTION

- Think honestly about your relationship with sex.
- Start conversations about sex with trusted friends and relatives.
- Pay attention to how sex affects your mood, emotions, and attitude when you're not in bed.
- Love your tree.
- Eat abundantly and creatively.
- Eat enough fat and cholesterol.
- Start addressing your issues now, not later.
- Practice forgiveness and self-love.
- Add love to your plate.

CONCLUSION

Seattle, Now

My life is vastly different than it was when I was a scared, hungry, abused little girl in Missouri, but it doesn't mean the challenges I face are much different than yours. I'm busy; between managing more than twenty Passionate Nutrition locations and their respective practitioners and juggling appearances, I've become very good at putting myself and my own needs last. It comes as no surprise that I'm most sexual on vacation, when my husband and I have a strict no-phone/no-Internet policy. (There is no better libido killer than a wireless connection.) At times, talking about nutrition nonstop makes me tend toward orthorexia, the third and often unknown major eating disorder, besides anorexia and bulimia, in which people develop an unhealthy obsession with eating well. That means that while I preach balance and the Living in the Gray Guideline (see page 53), I often have trouble adhering to it myself.

But today, I am also the best version of myself. I *love* who I am. And I think it's fascinating that along my path to the Jennifer of today, as I've added love and forgiveness to my life, I've thrown off many of the things that plagued me as a child and young adult beyond the illness I previously described—frigidity, fear, anger, shame, and embarrassment, to name a few. As I've grown my practice and watched others experience the same liberation, I've felt confident that the precepts described in this book work.

There's a spring that flows beneath the Tree of Hippocrates, in Kos, Greece—the tree under which Hippocrates himself, the father of medicine, is reported to have once taught his students. I sat there once—on our honeymoon in 2010—after Jon had called me "the medicine woman," because I'd recently told him about my past. He marveled at my ability to turn myself around. It didn't seem that outrageous to me, because I knew the power of food, and I'd learned the power of love. Together, the two make humans thrive. But under that tree, it occurred to me that if I could disseminate any of my learned wisdom on a grand scale, I might have some spot in humanity's centuries-long quest for health. I realized that being passionate about nutrition was, in fact, my calling. And if that's true—if I do have a place in that grand lineage, which I certainly don't take for granted—I have two goals: My first goal is to communicate that an enjoyable, long life starts with eating well, but only succeeds if we love well too. My second goal is to go out of business.

In that regard, this book, by definition, is about you. If I've succeeded, I've told you that I understand what life throws at us. My life's path is different from yours, but we are all, in some way, broken. We are an overbusy, sad, undernourished, angry, ashamed culture. But because we have access to food that can nourish us, and the ability, deep inside, to love ourselves, our bodies, and each other, we can heal.

Part IV

THE RECIPES

I f there is a single biggest misconception about cooking, it's that it needs to be difficult to be delicious and/or nutritious. I'm an expert at streamlining the cooking process, in part because I cook regularly, but mostly because I always take the simplest approach possible. Call it habit; years of living off the grid taught me that the simplest approach is often also the easiest. I don't peel anything but onions, garlic, and broccoli stems. I don't wash produce, knives, or cutting boards unless absolutely necessary and frequently leave cooked food out at room temperature for days. I use frozen, precut vegetables when I don't have much time. Whenever possible, I make double the amount I need and freeze or refrigerate extra portions for another meal. (A list posted on the refrigerator door helps me remember what's available and ready to eat.) I reuse dishes as much as possible—for example, I'll often use the same spoon to stir everything on the stove, if I have multiple pots going at once—and store leftovers in the vessel in which they were cooked and served, instead of transferring food from container to container. Generally, when dinner hits the table, I have one knife, one cutting board, and one pan to wash.

The following are my recipes, but if I were standing next to you in the kitchen, I'd probably tell you not to follow them. Cooking is instinctual. If you haven't done a lot of it, that can be a little scary, but know that your taste buds are always right. Personally, I often think food needs more salt and acid (usually in the form of vinegar) but not everyone tastes food the same way. Cook things the way you like them.

Note that the salt called for in these recipes is finely ground sea salt, not kosher or iodized salt. If you use kosher salt, decrease the amount by about 30 percent. I don't recommend using iodized salt.

DRINKS

Switchel (Ginger Elixer)

10 minutes active time / Makes 4 servings

This is a spinoff of a traditional switchel, a beverage with conflicting origins. Some believe it came from the Amish tradition, whereas others credit the West Indies; it may even date back to the time of Hippocrates, when water, vinegar, and honey were combined to make a medicinal drink. In any case, it's a good digestion enhancer, which means it's okay to drink with meals, and it helps the body absorb water. (I often prescribe it to people who say water goes right through them.) Feel free to adjust the proportions to suit your taste. To make ginger juice, use a Microplane or grater to grate the ginger, then squeeze the juice out of the ginger pulp with your hand.

If you'd like, garnish the drink with mint leaves or fresh berries.

- 4 cups water
- ¼ cup honey
- ¼ cup unpasteurized apple cider vinegar
- ¼ cup lemon juice
- 2½ tablespoons ginger juice
- ½ teaspoon sea salt

• In a large pitcher, combine the water and honey and whisk until blended. (If you have especially thick or cold honey, combine 1 cup of the water with the honey in a saucepan over low heat, dissolve it there, and then pour that dissolved mixture back into the pitcher.) Stir in the apple cider vinegar, lemon and ginger juices, and salt, whisking until the salt is completely dissolved, and serve warm, cool, or at room temperature. Refrigerate leftovers for up to 2 weeks.

Nettle Infusion

5 minutes active time / Makes 4 servings

Popularized by herbal healing expert Susun Weed, a nettle infusion is a great way for people who aren't absorbing nutrients well to get sufficient minerals. Because the water sits on the cell walls for hours, breaking them down, you get about 2,900 milligrams of calcium out of this infusion. Look for dried nettles in the bulk spice or tea aisle of large grocery stores or natural foods markets. I often make this before bed so it's ready in the morning.

....

1 ounce (about 1 cup, or a big handful) dried nettle leaves

½ cup dried peppermint leaves
4 cups cold water

....

- In a large pitcher, combine the nettles, peppermint, and water, stirring to submerge the leaves. Let sit at room temperature for 4 to 12 hours, strain through a fine-mesh strainer, and serve at room temperature. (You can also use a large French press to infuse the water without having to strain the leaves.) Refrigerate any leftover infusion for up to 1 week.

> **Note:** If desired, you can add cream, honey, vanilla, salt, or even vodka to taste. The goal is just get it in.

SNACKS

Crudités with Kimchi Cream Cheese Dip

5 minutes active time / Makes 1 heaping cup

Not everyone likes kimchi straight, which is why when I help people start incorporating it into their diet, I often give it a little bit of a disguise. Blended into cream cheese, it makes a dip as addictive as the packaged soup mix dips of our youth. If you don't have a food processor, just mash all the ingredients together with a fork. It won't be as smooth, but it's just as effective.

Since this travels well (and tastes great at room temperature), it's a good go-to snack to leave in the fridge at work or bring on trips.

8 ounces cream cheese (cultured, if possible), at room temperature

½ cup unpasteurized kimchi (with juice)

1 teaspoon sea salt

Cut raw vegetables, such as cucumbers, carrots, celery, radishes, cauliflower, jicama, broccoli, or snap peas, for serving

- In the work bowl of a food processor, pulse the cream cheese, kimchi, and salt until smooth. Serve with the vegetables or transfer to a sealable container and refrigerate for up to 2 months.

Change It Up:

- Stir in 1 cup fresh crabmeat or drained, canned crabmeat. Transfer to a small baking dish, bake at 350 degrees F for 10 minutes, and serve as an appetizer at room temperature, topped with additional kimchi. (You'll lose the dip's original beneficial bacteria, but it tastes great.)

- Add ½ cup cream and use as a dip for artichokes or a sauce for grilled chicken or salmon.

Crackers with Sardine-Olive Tapenade

15 minutes active time / Makes 4 to 6 servings

I happen to love eating sardines straight from their tin, but for some people who are new to them, they're best heaped on crackers, rolled into wraps, or piled onto a piece of toast. Sardines are one of the best sources of omega-3 fatty acids, with the added benefit of being much less expensive than fish like salmon.

1 garlic clove

1 (6-ounce) jar pitted kalamata olives, drained (about 1½ cups olives)

1 tablespoon capers

6 fresh basil leaves

⅓ cup extra-virgin olive oil

⅓ cup chopped piquillo peppers or roasted red bell peppers

2 (4-ounce) tins sardines, drained

¼ teaspoon freshly ground black pepper

Crackers, for serving

- In the work bowl of a food processor, add the garlic with the machine running and process until chopped. Add the olives and capers and pulse a few times, until finely chopped. Add the basil and pulse a few more times. Add the oil, peppers, and sardines, season with pepper, and pulse to your desired consistency. (If you don't have a food processor, you can just chop everything up very finely.) Serve on crackers at room temperature or transfer to a sealable container and refrigerate for up to 1 week.

Change It Up

- To make this more of a meal than a snack, fold in a can of drained, rinsed white beans and a handful of chopped parsley, then serve the salad on arugula dressed with Basic Apple Cider Vinaigrette (page 240).

Simple Chicken Liver Pâté

30 minutes active time / Makes 8 large servings

Liver is an excellent source of vitamins A, D, and B complex, as well as selenium, zinc, and iron, to name a few, but it's not something Americans are accustomed to eating nowadays. Simmered with onions, garlic, and white wine and blended with butter, it becomes a delicacy people dig (especially kids).

I chill my pâté in individual 8-ounce jars that I buy at the hardware store so I can take it with me to work easily. I eat it straight from the jar with crackers for a midmorning snack. If you'd like to get fancy, you can serve it at a party with toasts, Dijon mustard, and sea salt.

1½ cups (3 sticks) butter, at room temperature, divided

1 medium onion, thinly sliced

1 pound chicken livers, any liquid drained

⅓ cup white wine

1 tablespoon chopped fresh thyme, or 1 teaspoon dried thyme

1 large clove garlic, peeled and smashed

1 teaspoon sea salt

¼ teaspoon freshly ground black pepper

1 tablespoon unpasteurized apple cider vinegar

- In a large skillet over medium heat, melt ¼ cup (½ stick) of the butter. Add the onion, and cook, stirring occasionally, until completely soft, 10 to 15 minutes.

- Add the livers, wine, thyme, garlic, salt, and pepper to the pan, stir to combine, then bring the liquid to a simmer. Reduce the heat to cook at a low simmer for 6 to 8 minutes, until the livers are totally cooked on the outside but still a bit pink in the center, turning them occasionally to place the pinkest sides down in the pan. (The livers' shape and size will determine how long they take to cook.) Remove the pan from the heat and let cool for 5 minutes.

- Transfer the contents of the pan (including the liquid) to the work bowl of a food processor or blender and whirl until smooth. Add ¾ cup

(1½ sticks) of the butter to the food processor or blender, and whirl again until no clumps of butter remain. Add the vinegar, and whirl again, just until combined.

• Transfer the pâté to 8 small ramekins or 8-ounce glass jars and use a spoon or small knife to smooth down the tops. In a small pan over low heat, melt the remaining ½ cup (1 stick) of butter, and let cool for a few minutes. Carefully pour the butter over the top of the pâté in each container, so it just covers the top. (Although it's not necessary, this prevents the pâté from turning brown on top.) Let the pâté cool to room temperature, then refrigerate it for at least 4 hours before serving, and up to 2 weeks. (The butter acts as a sealant, so there's really no need to cover it.) Or the pâtés can be frozen, covered, for 3 to 6 months. In either case, it tastes best if you bring it to room temperature before serving.

Basic Egg Salad

15 minutes active time / Makes 4 to 6 servings

Eggs are considered the perfect protein. That they're versatile and economical is an added bonus; stirred into egg salad, they're good for snacks or lunches that are infinitely variable. When I make egg salad over the weekend, I separate it into a bunch of different snack containers and flavor each one differently, so I have a nutritious, totally prepared snack that tastes different each day. Typically, I bring it to work with me along with sliced jicama, cucumbers, or bell peppers, which all make good scoops.

....

1 dozen hard-cooked large eggs, peeled	1½ teaspoons sea salt
1½ cups sour cream	½ teaspoon freshly ground black pepper

....

• In a large bowl, smash the eggs with the side of a fork or a pastry cutter until they break into small pieces. Mix in the sour cream, salt, and pepper, then serve or transfer to a sealable container and refrigerate for up to 1 week.

continued

223

Change It Up:

- Add ¼ cup chopped fresh dill, tarragon, parsley, or basil.

- Add 3 tablespoons Dijon mustard.

- Add 2 tablespoons basil pesto or some of the pesto from the Roasted Salmon with Nettle Walnut Pesto (page 229).

- Add ½ cup salsa and ¼ cup chopped fresh cilantro.

- Add 1 tablespoon curry powder.

- Add ¼ cup prepared mole sauce.

Apple-Walnut Chicken Salad

15 minutes active time / Makes 4 to 6 servings

Packed with the right combination of fat, protein, and vital nutrients, this chicken salad is great for a snack or midday meal. You can buy a store-bought rotisserie chicken to save time or roast an extra chicken if you're making Roast Chicken with a Stick of Butter (page 230).

3 cups cooked chicken, coarsely chopped	1 large unpeeled apple, cored and coarsely chopped
1 cup toasted walnuts, coarsely chopped	1 cup sour cream
1 cup packed fresh basil, coarsely chopped	3 tablespoons lemon juice (from 1 large lemon)
3 stalks celery, coarsely chopped	1 teaspoon sea salt
	½ teaspoon freshly ground black pepper

- In a large sealable container, mix all the ingredients together until well blended. Serve immediately or refrigerate for up to 1 week.

MAINS

Miso Soup with Eggs and Mushrooms

30 minutes active time / Makes 4 servings

When you purchase Japanese miso paste, you can choose whichever one you're drawn to in the grocery store, but know that the darker the miso's color, the stronger a flavor it has. (Dark miso pastes are also more medicinal.) Remember that since any beneficial bacteria die when they get overheated, it's important to stir the miso in only once the soup has cooled enough to stick your finger into it comfortably.

....

½ cup toasted sesame oil

12 ounces crimini mushrooms, sliced (about 5 cups)

2 tablespoons sesame seeds

4 cups chicken stock (such as the Bone Broth on page 241)

8 large eggs

¼ cup *ume* plum vinegar

1 tablespoon miso paste

7 small scallions (everything but the root), sliced thinly on the diagonal, for garnish

....

- In a medium skillet over medium heat, add the oil, then the mushrooms, and stir until all the mushrooms are coated with the oil. Cook the mushrooms until they release their liquid, the liquid evaporates, and a deep-brown color develops, 20 to 25 minutes, stirring frequently. Add the sesame seeds and sauté for 1 to 2 minutes to toast them.

- While the mushrooms cook, make the soup: In a medium pot over medium-high heat, heat the chicken stock until it simmers. Reduce the heat to low, then, working quickly, crack the eggs into the pot one at a time. Whisk the soup vigorously after each addition to break up the egg white and yolk. Once all the eggs have been added, stir in the mushrooms, including all the good stuff left at the bottom of the pan. Remove the pan from the heat.

continued

- When the liquid is cool enough for you to stick your finger into comfortably, whisk in the vinegar and miso paste. (It is often easier to whisk the miso into a small amount of soup in a separate bowl, and then add it to the larger pot of soup.) Serve immediately in big bowls, garnished with the scallions.

> **Note:** Look for *ume* plum vinegar (also called *umeboshi* vinegar) in the ethnic foods aisle at a large grocery store or natural foods market.

Change It Up

- Before you remove the pot from the stove, stir in a handful of leftover chicken or steak.

- While the stock simmers, add about 2 dozen clams or mussels. Cover the pot and let the shellfish steam open for about 5 minutes, then remove the shellfish, discarding any that refuse to open. Finish making the soup, then add the shellfish back in before serving.

- Add leftover rice or other cooked grains, or leftover cooked vegetables, such as the vegetables from the Roast Chicken with a Stick of Butter (page 230).

Manila Clams with Wine, Butter, and Nettles

25 minutes active time / Makes 4 servings

In the spring, when nettles are fresh, I can't think of a more simple and satisfying way to end a day foraging than throwing the nettles' leaves into a pot of clams, where they release their earthy, herby flavor into the broth. If you don't have access to fresh nettles, use about 2 tablespoons of dried or substitute spinach, kale, or arugula.

You can also add a pinch of powdered seaweed to this recipe when you add the nettles.

2 pounds Manila clams	2 cups dry white wine
½ cup (1 stick) butter, divided	½ teaspoon sea salt
3 cloves garlic, finely chopped	Zest of 1 large lemon
¼ pound fresh nettles	

- In a large bowl, place the clams, add cold water to cover, and let sit for 15 minutes. (This allows the clams to spit out any extra sand they might have inside.) Drain and rinse the clams, discarding any that are broken or refuse to close, and set them aside.

- In a large, deep pot with a lid, melt ¼ cup (½ stick) of the butter over medium heat. Add the garlic and sauté for 1 minute. Using tongs, transfer the nettles to the pot, using kitchen scissors to trim them into 2-inch pieces as you go. Add the wine, increase the heat to high, and simmer for 5 minutes, stirring occasionally. Add the clams, stir to coat the clams in the sauce, cover the pot, and cook until all of the clams have opened, about 5 minutes. (Discard any clams that refuse to open.)

- Add the remaining ¼ cup (½ stick) of butter, salt, and lemon zest, stir to melt the butter, and serve the clams hot in wide, shallow bowls.

Mussels with Tomato Cream

25 minutes active time / Makes 4 servings

High in zinc and minerals, mussels are nutritional powerhouses hidden behind those beautiful shells. In the Pacific Northwest, I think we sometimes take them for granted; because they're inexpensive and easy to cook, it would be easy to make them staples on the dinner table in most households.

continued

Using the amount of red pepper flakes called for below gives the dish just a little bite; increase the amount to 1 or 1½ teaspoons if you want a broth that's truly spicy.

2 pounds mussels, such as Penn Cove

2 tablespoons butter

½ medium yellow onion, thinly sliced

2 cloves garlic, finely chopped

2 teaspoons chopped fresh thyme or oregano, or ½ teaspoon dried thyme or oregano

¼ to ½ teaspoon red pepper flakes

½ teaspoon powdered kelp or other seaweed (optional)

1 (14-ounce) can crushed tomatoes

¾ cup dry red wine

1 teaspoon sea salt

1 cup heavy cream

- In a large bowl, place the mussels, add cold water to cover, and let sit for 15 minutes. (This allows the mussels to spit out any extra sand they might have inside.) Drain and rinse the mussels, discarding any that are broken or refuse to close, and set them aside. (If the mussels have byssus threads, known as "beards," the stringy things that anchor them to their underwater homes, you can remove them by pulling on them perpendicular to the shell. They're fine to eat, but they have a texture some people find objectionable.)

- In a large, deep pot with a lid, melt the butter over medium heat. Add the onion and sauté for 3 minutes, or until the onion begins to soften. Add the garlic, thyme, red pepper flakes, and seaweed, and cook for 1 to 2 minutes more, stirring occasionally. Add the tomatoes, wine, and salt, increase the heat to high, and simmer for 10 minutes, stirring occasionally. Add the mussels, stir to coat the mussels in the sauce, cover the pot, and cook until all of the mussels have opened, about 5 minutes. (Discard any mussels that refuse to open.)

- Remove the pot from the heat and let rest for about a minute. Stir in the cream, then serve the mussels hot in wide, shallow bowls.

Change It Up

- Use white wine instead of red wine.

- Substitute a 14-ounce can of coconut milk for the wine and cream, and stir in the juice of a lime and 2 tablespoons grated ginger at the end.

Roasted Salmon with Nettle-Walnut Pesto

15 minutes active time / Makes 4 to 6 servings

The easiest way to preserve nettles when you find them in the wild in the spring—something I teach in my wild-foods foraging classes on the islands near Seattle—is to make pesto, which freezes beautifully. Use the pesto portion of this recipe to top the salmon or make a double or triple (or quadruple!) batch, and keep it for later, up to a month or longer in the refrigerator. I love having a jar in the refrigerator or freezer so that I can add it to chicken salad, mix it with sour cream for a quick raw-vegetable dip or sandwich spread, or mix it with a little more olive oil and use it as a sauce for grilled vegetables.

Nettles do sting, so handle them with gloves. Some people like to clean them or pick the leaves off one by one, but I typically pick them or buy them in a bag, and they get dumped directly from the bag into a pot of water. Like anything that grows in the wild, they might come with a stray bug or some dirt, but I'm not too concerned with that.

FOR THE PESTO:
¼ pound fresh nettles or ¼ cup cried nettles
1 clove garlic, peeled and smashed
¾ cup toasted walnuts
1 teaspoon sea salt
1 cup extra-virgin olive oil

1 loosely packed cup grated fresh Parmesan cheese
3 tablespoons lemon juice (from 1 large lemon)

1 (1½-pound) fillet wild salmon (such as sockeye, coho, or king)
½ teaspoon sea salt

- Preheat the oven to 425 degrees F.

continued

- If using dried nettles, place them in a bowl with ⅓ cup water and set aside.

- To make the pesto, fill a large pot with about 1½ inches of water. Bring the water to a boil, then add the nettles (strain if soaking dried nettles), stirring until they start to wilt, about 1 to 2 minutes. Cover and cook for 5 minutes, then drain. When the nettles have cooled enough to touch, squeeze out as much water as possible and set them aside.

- In the work bowl of a food processor, add the garlic and process until the garlic is finely chopped. Add the walnuts and pulse about 10 times, until finely chopped. Add the nettles, lemon juice, salt, and oil, and whirl until smooth. Add the Parmesan cheese and pulse just a few times. Transfer all but ½ cup of the pesto to a sealable container for other uses.

- Put the salmon in a roasting pan or on a baking sheet. Season it with the salt, then smear the reserved ½ cup pesto in an even layer all over the fillet.

- Roast the salmon for 10 to 15 minutes, or until you just begin to see small beads of white fat at the edges. Serve hot.

Change It Up:

- Grill the salmon. A 1½-pound fillet that's 1 inch thick, which is about right for 4 people, will take 10 to 15 minutes at 425 degrees F. Leave the lid closed so the top of the salmon cooks also.

Roast Chicken with a Stick of Butter

20 minutes active time / Serves 4 to 6

I think of roasting a chicken as the starting point to my week. Often, I roast two—you'll see this recipe is flexible. I use one for dinner that night, have enough leftover meat to make Apple-Walnut Chicken Salad (page 224), then I use the other to make some sort of Mexican chicken dish, like tacos or enchiladas, or a chicken soup. (One chicken usually yields about 4 cups of chopped meat, and that's if you don't clean it too meticulously.) I use the bones to make Bone Broth (page 241).

Note that what size you cut the vegetables isn't so important here and really, any combination of root vegetables works. The goal is to get something in the oven quickly, which is part of why I rarely wash or peel anything, and to provide something that soaks up all the chicken's delicious juices as it roasts. It's also why I never trim or tie my chickens.

Yes, you read right. An entire stick of butter. If you're roasting two chickens, use an additional ¼ cup (½ stick) butter and an additional teaspoon of salt to season the second bird.

....

6 carrots, cut into 2-inch pieces

2 red beets, cut into quarters

2 parsnips, turnips, and/or rutabagas, cut into 2-inch pieces

1 medium yellow onion, cut into eighths

5 cloves garlic, peeled and smashed

½ cup (1 stick) unsalted butter, at room temperature, divided

2 teaspoons sea salt, divided

½ to 1 teaspoon freshly ground black pepper, divided

1 or 2 (5-pound) chickens, giblets removed, patted dry with paper towels

2 tablespoons chopped fresh rosemary or thyme, or 2 teaspoons dried rosemary or thyme

....

- Preheat the oven to 450 degrees F.

- On the bottom of a roasting pan or a deep, rimmed baking sheet, spread the carrots, beets, parsnips, onions, and garlic. (If you're only roasting one chicken, a big cast iron pan works nicely too.) Cut ¼ cup (½ stick) of the butter into pieces and scatter them over the vegetables, then season the vegetables with half the salt and pepper. Place the chicken on top of the vegetables, breast side up, and rub the remaining ¼ cup (½ stick) of butter all over the skin. Season the chicken with the remaining salt and pepper. Sprinkle the rosemary over everything.

- Roast for about 1 hour, rotating the chicken 180 degrees about halfway if you happen to remember, or until the legs wiggle freely and an instant-read thermometer stuck in the thickest part of the thigh measures 165 degrees F. Let the chicken rest on the counter for about 10 minutes before cutting and serving.

A Mean Meat Loaf

25 minutes active time / Makes 4 servings

My first love, Suzanna, taught me to make a mean meat loaf. This version, made with grass-fed beef, is a great dinner, but in my house, we tend to eat it cold as a snack. Serve it over toast, cooked grains, or Parsnip Puree (page 239) for dinner, or pan-fry fat slices of it and top them with eggs for breakfast.

I like the flavor combination of fennel and red pepper flakes, but feel free to omit them if you'd prefer. Since meat loaf is infinitely variable, you can also stir in a handful of cooked, chopped vegetables or grains, or add ¼ pound ground organ meats to the mixture. The latter is my favorite variation, because it means I can get organ meats into the kids' diets without them noticing.

2 tablespoons butter, plus more for greasing the pan

1 medium onion, finely chopped

4 cloves garlic, minced

1 tablespoon chopped fresh thyme or oregano, or 1 teaspoon dried thyme or oregano

1 pound grass-fed ground beef

3 large eggs

¾ cup rolled oats

1 (6-ounce) can tomato paste, plus 1 (8-ounce) can tomato paste, for glaze

¼ cup chopped fresh parsley

1 tablespoon Dijon mustard

1 teaspoon sea salt

1 teaspoon powdered kelp or other seaweed

½ teaspoon red pepper flakes or freshly ground black pepper

½ teaspoon whole fennel seed, finely chopped

- Preheat the oven to 350 degrees F. Generously grease an 8-by-4-inch loaf pan with butter and set aside.

- In a large skillet over medium heat melt the butter. Add the onion and cook, stirring occasionally, for 10 minutes, or until the onion begins to brown. Add the garlic and thyme and cook for another 2 minutes, stirring once or twice.

- While the onion cooks, in a large bowl, mix together the beef, eggs, oats, 6 ounces of the tomato paste, parsley, mustard, salt, seaweed, red pepper flakes, and fennel. (I find using my hands works best.) Add the onion mixture, and stir to combine.

• Put the meat into the prepared pan, patting it into a roughly flat layer. Spoon the remaining 8 ounces of tomato paste over the top and bake for 45 to 50 minutes, or until the sauce is thick and bubbling, and the meat feels firm to the touch in the center.

• Let the meat loaf sit for 10 minutes before slicing and serving.

Wintry Spiced Beef Stew

30 minutes active time / Makes 4 servings

When you're feeding a family, buying grass-fed meat can get expensive, which is why I often cook with cheaper cuts such as stew meat and roasts. I find this stew convenient because it's made with ingredients that are either in the pantry or easy to freeze, which means it's something I can whip up at the end of a weekend away or at the end of the week without going grocery shopping again.

For variation, try substituting carrots, parsnips, or other root vegetables for the sweet potato. For instructions on how to make ginger juice, see the headnote in the Switchel (Ginger Elixer) recipe on page 218.

¼ cup (½ stick) butter or extra-virgin olive oil

1 pound grass-fed beef stew meat, cut into 1-inch squares

1 large onion, chopped

4 cloves garlic, minced

2 teaspoons smoked paprika

1 teaspoon ground cinnamon

¼ teaspoon freshly ground black pepper

¼ teaspoon cayenne pepper

½ cup prunes, chopped

1 bay leaf

3 cups chicken stock (such as the Bone Broth on page 241)

1 (14.5-ounce) can diced fire-roasted tomatoes

1 large unpeeled sweet potato, coarsely chopped, or 1 (10-ounce) bag frozen chopped sweet potatoes

2 teaspoons sea salt

1 teaspoon ginger juice

1 tablespoon lemon juice or unpasteurized apple cider vinegar

continued

- In a large soup pot over medium-high heat, melt the butter. Add the beef and cook, turning the pieces once or twice partway through when they release easily from the pan, for 8 to 10 minutes, or until all the beef pieces are nicely browned on 2 or 3 sides. Reduce the heat to medium and add the onions. Cook, stirring occasionally, another 10 minutes more, until the onions are soft. Stir in the garlic, paprika, cinnamon, pepper, cayenne, and prunes, and cook for 1 to 2 minutes, until the spices are fragrant. Add the bay leaf, stock, tomatoes, and sweet potatoes, and bring to a simmer. Reduce the heat to low and cook at a bare simmer for 1½ to 2 hours, or until the meat is totally tender. Remove and discard the bay leaf, season with the salt, add the ginger and lemon juices, and serve warm.

> **Note:** Instead of simmering the stew on the stove, you can transfer it, once you've added all the ingredients, to a slow cooker and cook on low heat for 6 to 8 hours.

SIDES

Asparagus with Creamy Miso Dressing

5 minutes active time / Makes 4 servings

Combining gut-friendly miso paste, which you'll find in the refrigerated section of most large grocery stores, with cream and ume *plum vinegar is a total crowd pleaser. Note that you can grill the asparagus, if you'd like. In that case, drizzle the sesame oil onto the asparagus before cooking, instead of after. Cook it on medium heat, at about 400 degrees F, for about 5 minutes, directly on the grates, turning the asparagus once or twice during cooking.*

··

1 pound asparagus, woody ends trimmed	1 tablespoon miso paste
	1 tablespoon *ume* plum vinegar
2 tablespoons heavy cream	1 tablespoon toasted sesame oil

··

- Heat about 1 inch of water in a large skillet over high heat. When the water simmers, add the asparagus, and cook for 3 to 5 minutes, depending on thickness, until the asparagus is bright green and tender in the center.

- Meanwhile, in a small bowl, stir together the cream, miso, and vinegar until smooth.

- Remove the asparagus with a slotted spoon and transfer it to a plate. Toss it with the sesame oil, then drizzle the miso sauce on top. Serve warm or at room temperature.

> **Note:** Look for *ume* plum vinegar (also called *umeboshi* vinegar) in the ethnic foods aisle at a large grocery store or natural foods market.

Change It Up:

- Substitute steamed, pan-fried, or grilled zucchini, carrots, bell peppers, broccoli, or cauliflower for the asparagus.

- Top the dish with toasted sesame seeds.

- Use the sauce on top of grilled chicken or fish.

Velvet Kale

25 minutes active time / Makes 4 servings

Consider this a gateway kale recipe. It's good for people focusing on gentle foods because the kale is well cooked; boiling it also removes some of its bitterness, which can turn people off. This is a great dish to have on hand to add to breakfasts—

continued

I serve it under a fried egg and top the egg with kimchi. Lacinato, or dinosaur kale, as it's sometimes called, is my favorite. If you're not a garlic lover, reduce the garlic to one or two cloves.

6 tablespoons (¾ stick) unsalted butter

1 large onion, halved and cut into ¼-inch-thick slices

1½ teaspoons sea salt

2 bunches (about 1 pound total) kale, stems removed

1 head garlic, chopped

2 tablespoons unpasteurized apple cider vinegar

- In a large skillet over medium-low heat, melt the butter. Add the onions, and cook, stirring every so often, until they have caramelized to a deep golden brown, 30 to 40 minutes or more. Season the onions with the salt.

- While the onions are cooking, bring a large pot of water to a boil, as if you're cooking pasta. Add the kale and let it boil, uncovered, for 10 minutes, stirring once or twice. Drain the kale, then use scissors to cut it into roughly 2-inch pieces.

- When the onions are brown, add the garlic and cook for 2 more minutes. Add the kale, and cook the mixture for 5 minutes, stirring occasionally. Remove the pan from the heat. Stir in the vinegar. Taste the kale, add more salt or vinegar if you want, and serve warm or at room temperature.

Massaged Kale and Currant Salad

15 minutes active time / Makes 6 servings

Besides being a delicious introduction to kale—the rock star of the produce aisle, if you ask me, because it's a nutrient powerhouse loaded with vitamins and minerals that boost energy—this salad is a go-to in my house because it tastes better the longer it sits. I often make a double batch, packing some in my lunch to make sure I get dark, leafy greens. It sounds crazy, but I think it's at its peak after about a week, and I keep it as long as two weeks in my refrigerator. If you can't find currants, raisins or dried cherries are also great.

1 large (about ¾ pound) bunch lacinato kale, stems removed, cut into bite-size pieces

1 teaspoon sea salt

¼ cup extra-virgin olive oil

2 tablespoons unpasteurized apple cider vinegar

¾ cup diced, unpeeled apple (about ½ medium apple)

⅓ cup currants

⅓ cup toasted sunflower seeds

¼ cup finely chopped red onion

⅓ cup crumbled Gorgonzola or feta cheese

- Put the kale in a large mixing bowl. Add the salt, and, using your hands, massage it into the kale for 2 minutes. Gently stir in the oil, vinegar, apple, currants, sunflower seeds, and onion. When all the ingredients are incorporated, gently stir in the cheese. Serve immediately, or refrigerate for up to 2 weeks.

Raw Beet Salad with Pumpkin Seeds and Parsley

10 minutes active time / Makes 6 to 8 servings

I'm a huge fan of vegetable salads that last longer than dinner does. Raw, grated beets are excellent candidates; paired with pumpkin seeds and parsley, they make a nutrient-packed crunchy salad that lasts for a good week in the refrigerator, getting better each day. Remember that you can also eat the green tops; chop them and sauté them in butter, then serve them with a good sprinkling of sea salt and a splash of apple cider vinegar. There's no need to peel the beets or apple.

3 medium (about 1 pound) red beets, grated

¼ cup unpasteurized apple cider vinegar

½ cup extra-virgin olive oil

1 cup toasted pumpkin seeds

1 Granny Smith apple, cored and grated or chopped

½ cup lightly packed chopped parsley

2 teaspoons sea salt

- In a large bowl, mix all the ingredients together. Serve immediately or refrigerate for up to 2 weeks (sometimes more, depending on your refrigerator).

continued

Change It Up:

• Substitute sesame seeds, sunflower seeds, or nuts for the pumpkin seeds.

• Add ¾ cup crumbled blue or feta cheese.

• Substitute chopped fresh dill, chives, basil, or tarragon for half of the parsley.

Simple Roasted Broccoli with Ume Plum Vinegar

5 minutes active time / Makes 4 servings

When I was a personal chef, I learned that when parents say their kids won't eat vegetables, roasted broccoli often breaks the ice. I discovered that the bright, tangy flavor of ume *plum vinegar made any food interesting. Note that a little goes a long way. If you're serving a crowd, double the recipe, but make sure you use a bigger pan (like a baking sheet) so the broccoli has room to roast instead of steam.*

2 tablespoons butter

1 pound broccoli, chopped into bite-size florets, stems peeled and chopped

½ teaspoon sea salt

2 teaspoons *ume* plum vinegar

• Preheat the oven to 450 degrees F.

• On a rimmed baking sheet in the oven, melt the butter. Put the broccoli on the baking sheet and toss with the butter and salt. Spread the broccoli out in a single layer. Bake until the broccoli is crunchy, dark brown, and almost burnt, about 20 to 30 minutes, depending on the size of the florets, stirring once halfway through the cooking. Remove from the oven, splash with the vinegar, toss, and serve.

> **Note:** Look for *ume* plum vinegar (also called *umeboshi* vinegar) in the ethnic foods aisle at a large grocery store or natural foods market.

Change It Up:

• Add a handful of toasted pine nuts or toasted walnuts when you add the vinegar.

• Instead of the vinegar, stir in a clove of finely chopped garlic and the juice of a lemon, plus a pinch more salt, after the first 10 minutes.

• Try using cauliflower instead of broccoli.

Parsnip Puree

15 minutes active time / Makes 8 to 10 servings

Root vegetables are loaded with minerals. They also carry with them the tenacious, persevering energy required to grow deep into hard soil, which is nutritious for the eater. I make this puree in abundance and heat it up for leftovers. Serve it under meat loaf, roasted chicken, or roast beef; alongside a fillet of fish; or for breakfast, with a poached egg and sautéed greens on top.

....

5 medium unpeeled parsnips, cut into big chunks (about 1 inch)

3 medium unpeeled potatoes, cut into big chunks (about 1 inch)

¼ cup (½ stick) butter

1½ cups heavy cream

1 tablespoon plus 1 teaspoon *ume* plum vinegar

1 tablespoon sea salt

2 teaspoons smoked paprika (also sold as *pimentón*)

....

• In a large pot, place the parsnips and potatoes and cover with water by about 1 inch. Bring to a boil over high heat and cook until a knife cuts through the vegetables with no resistance, 15 to 20 minutes. Drain the parsnips and potatoes. Return the pot to the stove over medium-low heat and add the butter. Put the hot parsnips and potatoes right on the butter and let them sit for a few minutes, so the heat from the vegetables melts the butter. Once the butter is melted, add the cream, vinegar, salt, and paprika.

continued

- Use an electric mixer or a potato masher to mash the vegetables until they are the consistency you like (or transfer them to a stand mixer fitted with the paddle attachment and whip on medium speed until pureed). Serve hot or at room temperature.

> **Note:** Look for *ume* plum vinegar (also called *umeboshi* vinegar) in the ethnic foods aisle at a large grocery store or natural foods market.

STAPLES

Basic Apple Cider Vinaigrette

5 minutes active time / Makes 2 cups

If there's one vinaigrette to keep on hand, it's this. Make a habit of shaking up a batch on the weekends, so that when it comes time to whip up something quickly on a weeknight, you have it on hand. It's an easy, tasty way to incorporate raw apple cider vinegar into your diet. For variation, try stirring in ¼ cup heavy cream, 2 cloves of finely chopped garlic, and/or a handful of finely chopped fresh herbs.

I like my salad dressing pretty spunky. If this tastes too vibrant for you, add an additional tablespoon or two of olive oil.

1¼ cups extra-virgin olive oil
½ cup unpasteurized apple cider vinegar
1 tablespoon Dijon mustard
1 teaspoon sea salt
½ teaspoon freshly ground black pepper

- Put all the ingredients in a pint-size glass jar with a lid. Shake vigorously, until well combined. Use immediately or refrigerate the jar indefinitely, letting it come up to room temperature and shaking before using each time.

Quick Ideas for Basic Apple Cider Vinaigrette

- Drizzle it over a salad of arugula, pulled chicken, avocado, and walnuts.
- Stir it into a bowl of cooked white or garbanzo beans with olives, chopped tomato, red onion, herbs, and goat cheese.
- Use it to dress ½ pound each of thinly sliced radicchio and endive garnished with Italian parsley.
- Blend it with sour cream to create a dressing for tuna, chicken, or egg salad.
- Use it as a simple dressing for wild herbs like sorrel, chickweed, or dandelion, with a drizzle of honey added, if desired.

Bone Broth

30 minutes active time / Makes 4 quarts

Called bone broth, clear broth, chicken stock, or just plain magic, simmering water with chicken bones and aromatics makes a tonic that transforms health. In my version of bone broth, I add vinegar to help encourage the collagen out of the bones and kombu, a type of seaweed readily available in dried form, because, while it doesn't affect the taste of the stock, it adds a velvety texture and plenty of minerals.

If you are using this medicinally—to improve hair and skin or to calm and nourish your digestive system—aim to drink 1 to 3 cups per day, either straight (in which case it's nice to add sea salt and/or ume plum or apple cider vinegar) or in foods. For ease, I recommend refrigerating it in quart-size glass jars, which are easy to take to work and double as a drinking vessel so you can just take the lid off and reheat. I keep a hefty stash in the freezer but have some defrosted at all times.

Leaving the salt out of the original batch makes the broth more versatile; you can use it in place of water when cooking grains or beans or making soups. Apologize to the boxed chicken stock in your pantry; you may never use it again.

There is no need to peel any of the vegetables; just break them up, if necessary, so they fit into your pot.

continued

1 whole pastured chicken with bones (including the giblets, wings, neck, and back, if possible)

4 quarts water

3 stalks celery

2 carrots, broken just to fit in the pot

1 large onion (whole, skin and all)

2 tablespoons unpasteurized apple cider vinegar or lemon juice

1 (6-inch) piece kombu (dried seaweed), optional

1 bunch parsley

- In a large stainless steel pot, combine the chicken, water, celery, carrots, onion, vinegar, and seaweed, and bring to a boil over high heat. Reduce the heat to a low simmer and cook, covered, for 6 to 48 hours—the longer you cook the stock, the richer and more flavorful it will be. (If you prefer, you can remove the chicken after an hour or two, picking off the meat and reserving it for chicken salad, enchiladas, and other dishes, and then return the bones and anything else you will not eat back to the pot.)

- Let the stock cool, then strain it through a fine-mesh strainer, discarding the solids. Transfer it to sealable containers, and refrigerate it for up to 2 weeks or freeze it for up to 1 year.

Note: If you have time, break the chicken bones up with a large cleaver; the nutrients inside the bones are more easily incorporated into the stock that way. If you do this, the stock will probably be thick, like Jell-O, when it comes out of the refrigerator. This means the stock has plenty of gelatin, which is great for your body. (It will relax once you rewarm it.)

APPENDIX

Answer Key to
QUIZ: Do You Know Nutrition? (page 23)

1. **B—False**

   People who have tried to lose weight by eating less and exercising more eventually learn that this is a great way to feel bad about themselves. It's a flawed method. If it worked, we wouldn't struggle so much with losing and maintaining our natural weight. I discuss the factors that contribute to weight gain and loss in Chapter 6.

2. **B—False**

   Every single cell in our body needs fat. If we were to perform liposuction on the fat surrounding our entire body, we would die. Eating a diet of fat-free and low-fat foods is a great way to have dry skin and hair, and to acquire a drawn, aged look. Plus, when we don't eat enough fat, we are typically not very happy or fun to be around.

3. **B—False**

   Contrary to what most people believe, raw foods are not always more nutritious—many foods are more readily absorbed when they are cooked. (Nutritionists call this "bioavailability.") For example, if we eat a raw carrot, we only absorb about 3 percent of its beta-carotene, which is the nutrient carrots are known for. If we eat cooked carrots and fat, we absorb 39 percent of their beta-carotene. Also, did you know that sweet potatoes and kale have more beta-carotene than carrots?

4. **B—Potato**

   Of the foods listed, potatoes have the highest level of potassium per serving. An average baked potato (with the skin on) supplies 926 milligrams of potassium, or 26 percent of the Daily Value (DV). Most people associate high potassium with bananas, which can be attributed to one brilliant marketing campaign, yet a banana supplies us with less than half (422 milligrams, or 12 percent of the DV) of the potassium we get from a potato. You may be surprised to learn that even salmon has more potassium than bananas. Bananas are a leading source of potassium among fruits, but don't come close to providing the levels of potassium of many other foods.

5. **C—Seaweed**

This power food offers the broadest range of minerals of any food and contains practically all the minerals found in the ocean. Seaweed is rich in iodine, vitamin K, calcium, and even fiber. It can nourish your thyroid, which boosts metabolism, promotes longevity and digestive health, and brings more shine to your hair and skin. In Chapter 7, you'll find tips for adding seaweed to your diet in ways that taste good, and the recipe section of the book, which begins on page 215, offers dishes that include seaweed.

6. **B—False**

Without salt we cannot live, much less have dependably good health. The caveat is that it's important to choose unrefined salt. Refined salt, also known as table salt, is stripped of all its life-giving minerals during the manufacturing process. Unrefined salt (Celtic sea salt and Himalayan pink salt, for example) contains about eighty minerals and elements essential for life. Harvesters of unrefined salt rely on ancient methods to retain the salt's minerals, which help the body maintain a healthy pH balance and strengthen the immune system. We eat less salt today than at any other time in history. Surprised?

7. **E—C and D (red meat and dairy)**

Because of bioaccumulation, or the accumulation of a substance in a living organism, organic meat and dairy give you the biggest bang for your buck. Over its lifetime, a 1,000-pound cow consumes far more pesticides (which are added to its feed) than a carrot or strawberry would be capable of absorbing. A study in Israel found that when people consumed organic meat and dairy, they reduced their exposure to certain estrogen-related pesticides by 98 percent.

8. **B—False**

Saturated fats are not dangerous or to blame for heart disease. We need saturated fat to live. Our cells require it for structure and function. (See pages 176–177 for more information on saturated fats.) When it comes to saturated fat, most of us still rely on the results of outdated studies; many large, well-designed studies published in reputable medical journals do not support the association between saturated fat and heart disease.

9. **C—Sugar**

A pair of 2013 Connecticut College studies showed that the part of rats' brains that respond to pleasure—the same portion often studied in connected to addiction—responded more strongly to an Oreo at the end of a maze than they did to an injection of morphine or cocaine.

10. **E—All of the above**

Meat from grass-fed animals is lower in fat than meat from grain-fed animals, and it's also lower in calories. The average American consumed 64.4 pounds of beef a year in 2000, so switching to lean, grass-fed beef can save you more than 17,000 calories per year. That's a lot of calories for a pretty slight shift. If everything else in your diet remains constant, in theory you'll lose about six pounds a year. Plus, you receive the health benefits of higher omega-3 fatty acids (good for your mood, skin, and hair) and conjugated linoleic acid for help with cancer prevention.

11. **D—Bell peppers**

High in vitamin C and beta-carotene, bell peppers provide 195.8 percent of your DV of vitamin C. A half cup of raw red bell pepper contains more than 140 milligrams of vitamin C. All bell peppers are high in vitamin C, but yellow are the highest; red peppers come in second. If your first choice was oranges, you, like millions of others, have fallen prey to marketing. Papayas, bell peppers, broccoli, brussels sprouts, strawberries, and pineapple all have more vitamin C per serving than oranges.

12. **A—One avocado**

One avocado has 13 grams of fiber, while a slice of whole-wheat bread has 3 grams, a side garden salad has 4, and a large peach has 3. When I need a quick snack, I will cut an avocado in half, sprinkle it with salt, and eat the whole thing with a spoon.

RESOURCES

For Readers:

Bacon, Linda, PhD. *Health at Every Size: The Surprising Truth About Your Weight*. Dallas: Benbella, 2008.

Bailor, Jonathan. *The Calorie Myth: How to Eat More, Exercise Less, Lose Weight, and Live Better*. New York: HarperCollins, 2014.

Blaser, Martin J., MD. *Missing Microbes: How the Overuse of Antibiotics is Fueling Our Modern Plagues*. New York: Henry Holt, 2014.

Brownstein, David, MD. *Salt Your Way to Health*. 2nd ed. West Bloomfield, MI: Medical Alternative Press, 2006.

David, Marc. *Nourishing Wisdom: A Mind-Body Approach to Nutrition and Well-Being*. New York: Bell Tower, 1991.

-----. *The Slow Down Diet: Eating for Pleasure, Energy, and Weight Loss*. Rochester, VT: Healing Arts Press, 2005.

Ensler, Eve. *The Vagina Monologues*. New York: Villard, 1998.

Fallon, Sally. *Nourishing Traditions: The Cookbook that Challenges Politically Correct Nutrition and the Diet Dictocrats*. Washington, DC: NewTrends, 2001.

Fisher, Helen. *Why We Love: The Nature and Chemistry of Romantic Love*. New York: Owl, 2004.

Fromm, Erich. *The Art of Loving*. Fiftieth anniversary edition. New York: HarperCollins, 2006.

Gershon, Michael. *The Second Brain: A Groundbreaking New Understanding of Nervous Disorders of the Stomach and Intestine*. New York: HarperCollins, 1998.

Katie, Byron and Stephen Mitchell. *Loving What Is: Four Questions That Can Change Your Life*. New York: Three Rivers, 2002.

Katz, Sandor Ellix. *Wild Fermentation: The Flavor, Nutrition, and Craft of Live-Culture Foods*. White River Junction, VT: Chelsea Green, 2003.

Keys, Ancel Benjamin. *Seven Countries: A Multivariate Analysis of Death and Coronary Heart Disease*. Cambridge, MA: Harvard University Press, 1980.

Kurlansky, Mark. *Salt: A World History*. New York: Penguin, 2003.

Lair, Cynthia. *Feeding the Whole Family*. Seattle: Sasquatch, 2008.

Leach, Jeff. *Honor Thy Symbionts*. Jeff Leach, n.p.: printed by CreateSpace, 2012.

Miller, Daphne, MD. *The Jungle Effect: The Healthiest Diets from Around the World—Why They Work and How to Make Them Work for You*. New York: HarperCollins, 2009.

Myers, Eileen Stellefson, MPH, RDN, FADA. *Winning the War Within*. Lake Dallas, TX: Helm, 2008. Copyright 2008: Used by permission of Helm Publishing Inc.

Perlmutter, David, MD and Kristin Loberg. *Grain Brain: The Surprising Truth About Wheat, Carbs, and Sugar—Your Brain's Silent Killers*. New York: Little, Brown and Company, 2013.

Pollan, Michael. *Cooked: A Natural History of Transformation*. New York: Penguin, 2014.

Rankin, Lissa, MD. *Mind Over Medicine: Scientific Proof That You Can Heal Yourself*. Carlsbad, CA: Hay House, 2013.

Robinson, Jo. *Eating on the Wild Side: The Missing Link to Optimum Health*. New York: Little, Brown and Company, 2013.

Taubes, Gary. *Why We Get Fat: And What to Do About It*. New York: Knopf, 2011.

Tribole, Evelyn. *Intuitive Eating*. 3rd ed. New York: St. Martin's Griffin, 2012.

Wann, Marilyn. *FAT!SO?: Because You Don't Have to Apologize for Your Size*. Berkeley: Ten Speed, 1998.

Weed, Susun. *Breast Cancer? Breast Health! The Wise Woman Way*. Woodstock, NY: Ash Tree Publishing, 1996.

-----. *Down There: Sexual and Reproductive Health the Wise Woman Way*. Woodstock, NY: Ash Tree Publishing, 2011.

Great Online Resources:

Cynthia Lair
CynthiaLair.com

Daniel Vitalis: Rewild Yourself
DanielVitalis.com

Eat Wild: Getting Wild Nutrition from Modern Food
EatWild.com

Environmental Working Group
EWG.org

Ellyn Satter Institute
EllynSatterInstitute.org

Global Culture of Women
GlobalCultureOfWomen.org

Institute for the Psychology of Eating
PsychologyOfEating.com

Linus Pauling Institute at Oregon State University
LPI.OregonState.edu

Ryan Drum
RyanDrum.com

The Weston A. Price Foundation
WestonAPrice.org

BIBLIOGRAPHY
by CHAPTER

Chapter 2

Centers for Disease Control and Prevention. "CDC - Number of Persons - Diagnosed Diabetes - Data & Trends - Diabetes DDT." http://www.cdc.gov/diabetes/statistics/prev/national/figpersons.htm.

Daley, Cynthia A., Amber Abbott, Patrick S. Doyle, Glenn A. Nader, and Stephanie Larson. "A Review of Fatty Acid Profiles and Antioxidant Content in Grass-Fed and Grain-Fed Beef." *Nutrition Journal* 9, no. 1 (March 10, 2010): 10. doi:10.1186/1475-2891-9-10.

David, Marc. "The Missing Ingredient in Nutrition." 2014. http://psychologyofeating.com/the-missing-ingredient-in-nutrition/.

Pan American Health Organization. "Health Situation Analysis and Trends Summary: United States of America." http://www1.paho.org/English/DD/AIS/cp_840.htm.

Simopoulos, Artemis P., and J. M. Ordovas, eds. *Nutrigenetics and Nutrigenomics*. World Review of Nutrition and Dietetics, v. 93. Basel, Switzerland; New York: S. Karger, 2004.

United States Department of Agriculture. "Agricultural Fact Book 2001-2002." March 2003. http://www.usda.gov/documents/usda-factbook-2001-2002.pdf.

Wade, Nicholas. "Your Body Is Younger Than You Think." *New York Times*, August 2, 2005. http://www.nytimes.com/2005/08/02/science/02cell.html.

Chapter 3

Albritton, Jen. "Modernizing Your Diet With Traditional Foods." Weston A. Price Foundation. http://www.westonaprice.org/health-topics/modernizing-your-diet-with-traditional-foods/.

Amin, Mohamed, Duncan Willetts, and John Earnes. *Last of the Maasai*. London: Camerapix, 2004.

Aubrey, Allison. "The Full-Fat Paradox: Whole Milk May Keep Us Lean." NPR.org. http://www.npr.org/blogs/thesalt/2014/02/12/275376259/the-full-fat-paradox-whole-milk-may-keep-us-lean.

Bakalar, Nicholas. "Study Linking Illness and Salt Leaves Researchers Doubtful." *New York Times*, April 22, 2014. http://www.nytimes.com/2014/04/22/health/study-linking-illness-and-salt-leaves-researchers-doubtful.html.

Barlow, Tom. "Americans Cook the Least, Eat the Fastest." Forbes.com. http://www.forbes.com/sites/tombarlow/2011/04/15/americans-cook-the-least-eat-the-fastest/.

Benbrook, Charles M., Gillian Butler, Maged A. Latif, Carlo Leifert, and Donald R. Davis. "Organic Production Enhances Milk Nutritional Quality by Shifting Fatty Acid Composition: A United States–Wide, 18-Month Study." *PLOS ONE* 8, no. 12 (December 9, 2013): e82429. doi:10.1371/journal.pone.0082429.

Burns, Sarah. "Nutritional Value of Fruits, Veggies Is Dwindling." Msnbc.com. http://www.nbcnews.com/id/37396355/ns/health-diet_and_nutrition/t/nutritional-value-fruits-veggies-dwindling/.

Center for Food Safety and Applied Nutrition. "Ingredients, Additives, GRAS & Packaging - Guidance for Industry: Estimating Dietary Intake of Substances in Food." http://www.fda.gov/food/guidanceregulation/guidancedocumentsregulatoryinformation/ingredientsadditivesgraspackaging/ucm074725.htm#ingr.

Crewe, J. R. "The Milk Cure: Real Milk Cures Many Diseases." A Campaign for Real Milk. http://www.realmilk.com/health/milk-cure/.

Dixon, T., M. Shaw, S. Ebrahim, and P. Dieppe. "Trends in Hip and Knee Joint Replacement: Socioeconomic Inequalities and Projections of Need." *Annals of the Rheumatic Diseases* 63, no. 7 (July 1, 2004): 825–30. doi:10.1136/ard.2003.012724.

Duffey, Kiyah J., and Barry M. Popkin. "High-Fructose Corn Syrup: Is This What's for Dinner?" *American Journal of Clinical Nutrition* 88, no. 6 (December 1, 2008): 1722S–1732S. doi:10.3945/ajcn.2008.25825C.

Graudal, Niels, Gesche Jürgens, Bo Baslund, and Michael H. Alderman. "Compared With Usual Sodium Intake, Low- and Excessive-Sodium Diets Are Associated With Increased Mortality: A Meta-Analysis." *American Journal of Hypertension* (March 20, 2014): hpu028. doi:10.1093/ajh/hpu028.

Holmberg, Sara, and Anders Thelin. "High Dairy Fat Intake Related to Less Central Obesity: A Male Cohort Study with 12 Years' Follow-Up." *Scandinavian Journal of Primary Health Care* 31, no. 2 (June 2013): 89–94. doi:10.31 09/02813432.2012.757070.

Hu, Frank B. "Globalization of Diabetes The Role of Diet, Lifestyle, and Genes." *Diabetes Care* 34, no. 6 (June 1, 2011): 1249–57. doi:10.2337/dc11-0442.

Omar, Syed Haris. "Oleuropein in Olive and Its Pharmacological Effects." *Scientia Pharmaceutica* 78, no. 2 (2010): 133–54. doi:10.3797/scipharm. 0912-18.

Paula, Elle. "The Most Common Food Preservatives." Livestrong.com. http://www.livestrong.com/article/288335-the-most-common-food-preservatives/.

Philpott, Tom. "The American Diet in One Chart, with Lots of Fats and Sugars." Grist. http://grist.org/industrial-agriculture/2011-04-05-american-diet-one-chart-lots-of-fats-sugars/.

Robinson, Jo. "Breeding the Nutrition Out of Our Food." *New York Times*, May 25, 2013. http://www.nytimes.com/2013/05/26/opinion/sunday/breeding-the-nutrition-out-of-our-food.html.

Statistical Office of the European Communities. "How Europeans Spend Their Time Everyday Life of Women and Men." Luxembourg: Office for Official Publications of the European Commission, 2004. http://epp. eurostat.ec.europa.eu/cache/ITY_OFFPUB/KS-58-04-998/EN/KS-58-04-998-EN.PDF.

Taubes, Gary. "The (Political) Science of Salt." *Science* 281, no. 5379 (August 14, 1998): 898–907. doi:10.1126/science.281.5379.898.

"The Inuit Paradox—High Protein & Fat, No Fruits/Vegetables and yet Lower Heart Disease and Cancer." The IF Life. http://www.theiflife.com/the-inuit-paradox-high-fat-lower-heart-disease-and-cancer/.

Tremblay, Louise. "Nutrients That Help Build and Maintain Body Cells & Tissues." Livestrong.com. http://www.livestrong.com/article/321741-nutrients-that-help-build-and-maintain-body-cells-tissues/.

United States Department of Agriculture. "Nutrient Content of the U.S. Food Supply, 1909-2000." November 2004. http://www.cnpp.usda.gov/publications/foodsupply/FoodSupply1909-2000.pdf.

Chapter 4

Caporaso, J. Gregory, Christian L. Lauber, Elizabeth K. Costello, Donna Berg-Lyons, Antonio Gonzalez, Jesse Stombaugh, Dan Knights, et al. "Moving Pictures of the Human Microbiome." *Genome Biology* 12, no. 5 (2011): R50. doi:10.1186/gb-2011-12-5-r50.

Conly, J. M., and K. Stein. "The Production of Menaquinones (Vitamin K2) by Intestinal Bacteria and Their Role in Maintaining Coagulation Homeostasis." *Progress in Food & Nutrition Science* 16, no. 4 (December 1992): 307–43.

Grice, Elizabeth A., Heidi H. Kong, Sean Conlan, Clayton B. Deming, Joie Davis, Alice C. Young, Gerard G. Bouffard, et al. "Topographical and Temporal Diversity of the Human Skin Microbiome." *Science* 324, no. 5931 (May 29, 2009): 1190–92. doi:10.1126/science.1171700.

Kresser, Chris. "Kefir: The Not-Quite-Paleo Superfood." http://chriskresser.com/kefir-the-not-quite-paleo-superfood.

LeBlanc, Jean Guy, Christian Milani, Graciela Savoy de Giori, Fernando Sesma, Douwe van Sinderen, and Marco Ventura. "Bacteria as Vitamin Suppliers to Their Host: A Gut Microbiota Perspective." *Current Opinion in Biotechnology* 24, no. 2 (April 2013): 160–68. doi:10.1016/j.copbio.2012.08.005.

Liou, Alice P., Melissa Paziuk, Jesus-Mario Luevano, Sriram Machineni, Peter J. Turnbaugh, and Lee M. Kaplan. "Conserved Shifts in the Gut Microbiota Due to Gastric Bypass Reduce Host Weight and Adiposity." *Science Translational Medicine* 5, no. 178 (March 27, 2013): 178ra41–178ra41. doi:10.1126/scitranslmed.3005687.

Noh, Jeong Sook, Hyun Ju Kim, Myung Ja Kwon, and Yeong Ok Song. "Active Principle of Kimchi, 3-(4-Hydroxyl-3,5-Dimethoxyphenyl)propionic

Acid, Retards Fatty Streak Formation at Aortic Sinus of Apolipoprotein E Knockout Mice." *Journal of Medicinal Food* 12, no. 6 (December 1, 2009): 1206–12. doi:10.1089/jmf.2009.0034.

Pollan, Michael. "Say Hello to the 100 Trillion Bacteria That Make Up Your Microbiome." *New York Times Magazine*, May 15, 2013. http://www.nytimes.com/2013/05/19/magazine/say-hello-to-the-100-trillion-bacteria-that-make-up-your-microbiome.html.

Ramakrishna, B. S. "Role of the Gut Microbiota in Human Nutrition and Metabolism." *Journal of Gastroenterology and Hepatology*, 28 (2013): 9–17. doi: 10.1111/jgh.12294.

Rao, A. Venket, Alison C. Bested, Tracey M. Beaulne, Martin A. Katzman, Christina Iorio, John M. Berardi, and Alan C. Logan. "A Randomized, Double-Blind, Placebo-Controlled Pilot Study of a Probiotic in Emotional Symptoms of Chronic Fatigue Syndrome." *Gut Pathogens* 1, no. 1 (2009): 6. doi:10.1186/1757-4749-1-6.

Ridaura, Vanessa K., Jeremiah J. Faith, Federico E. Rey, Jiye Cheng, Alexis E. Duncan, Andrew L. Kau, Nicholas W. Griffin, et al. "Gut Microbiota from Twins Discordant for Obesity Modulate Metabolism in Mice." *Science* 341, no. 6150 (September 6, 2013): 1241214. doi:10.1126/science.1241214.

Rook, Graham A. W., and Christopher A. Lowry. "The Hygiene Hypothesis and Psychiatric Disorders." *Trends in Immunology* 29, no. 4 (April 2008): 150–58. doi:10.1016/j.it.2008.01.002.

Taylor, Marygrace. "A New Weight Loss Elixir?" *Prevention*. http://www.prevention.com/weight-loss/weight-loss-tips/how-apple-cider-vinegar-could-slim-you-down.

Watanabe, Hiromitsu. "Beneficial Biological Effects of Miso with Reference to Radiation Injury, Cancer and Hypertension." *Journal of Toxicologic Pathology* 26, no. 2 (June 2013): 91–103. doi:10.1293/tox.26.91.

Weed, Susun. "Optimum Nutrition Cooked or Raw." 2004. http://www.susunweed.com/herbal_ezine/april04/healingwise.htm.

Young, Simon N. "How to Increase Serotonin in the Human Brain without Drugs." *Journal of Psychiatry & Neuroscience* 32, no. 6 (November 2007): 394–99.

Chapter 5

Elango, Rajavel, Mohammad A. Humayun, Ronald O. Ball, and Paul B. Pencharz. "Evidence That Protein Requirements Have Been Significantly Underestimated." *Current Opinion in Clinical Nutrition and Metabolic Care* 13, no. 1 (January 2010): 52–57. doi:10.1097/MCO.0b013e328332f9b7.

Jaslow, Ryan. "World Health Organization Lowers Sugar Intake Recommendations." CBS News. http://www.cbsnews.com/news/world-health-organization-lowers-sugar-intake-recommendations/.

Kniskern, Megan A., and Carol S. Johnston. "Protein Dietary Reference Intakes May Be Inadequate for Vegetarians If Low Amounts of Animal Protein Are Consumed." *Nutrition* 27, no. 6 (June 2011): 727–30. doi:10.1016/j.nut.2010.08.024.

Pappas, Stephanie. "Oreos Are as Enticing as Cocaine, a Rat Study Finds. But Don't Worry about Withdrawal." *Washington Post*, October 21, 2013. http://wapo.st/1c22NkU.

Soechtig, Stephanie. *Fed Up.* Documentary film. Santa Monica, CA: Atlas Films, 2014.

World Health Organization. "Protein and Amino Acid Requirements in Human Nutrition." WHO Technical Report Series 935, 2007. http://www.who.int/nutrition/publications/nutrientrequirements/WHO_TRS_935/en/.

Chapter 6

ABC News. "100 Million Dieters, $20 Billion: The Weight-Loss Industry by the Numbers." ABC News online, May 14, 2012. http://abcnews.go.com/Health/100-million-dieters-20-billion-weight-loss-industry/story?id=16297197.

Ahmad, Jamal, Faiz Ahmed, Mohammad A. Siddiqui, Basharat Hameed, and Ibne Ahmad. "Inflammation, Insulin Resistance and Carotid IMT in First Degree Relatives of North Indian Type 2 Diabetic Subjects." *Diabetes Research and Clinical Practice* 73, no. 2 (August 2006): 205–10. doi:10.1016/j.diabres.2006.01.009.

Ahmed, Abeer A., Kayode A. Balogun, Natalia V. Bykova, and Sukhinder K. Cheema. "Novel Regulatory Roles of Omega-3 Fatty Acids in Metabolic Pathways: A Proteomics Approach." *Nutrition & Metabolism* 11, no. 1 (January 17, 2014): 6. doi:10.1186/1743-7075-11-6.

Chowdhury, Rajiv, Samantha Warnakula, Setor Kunutsor, Francesca Crowe, Heather A. Ward, Laura Johnson, Oscar H. Franco, et al. "Association of Dietary, Circulating, and Supplement Fatty Acids With Coronary Risk: A Systematic Review and Meta-Analysis." *Annals of Internal Medicine* 160, no. 6 (March 18, 2014): 398–406. doi:10.7326/M13-1788.

Henig, Robin Marantz. "Fat Factors." *New York Times Magazine*, August 13, 2006. http://www.nytimes.com/2006/08/13/magazine/13obesity.html.

Huerta, Milagros G., James N. Roemmich, Marit L. Kington, Viktor E. Bovbjerg, Arthur L. Weltman, Viola F. Holmes, James T. Patrie, Alan D. Rogol, and Jerry L. Nadler. "Magnesium Deficiency Is Associated With Insulin Resistance in Obese Children." *Diabetes Care* 28, no. 5 (May 1, 2005): 1175–81. doi:10.2337/diacare.28.5.1175.

Hyman, Mark. "The Key to Automatic Weight Loss!" http://drhyman.com/blog/2014/05/19/key-automatic-weight-loss/.

Kresser, Chris. "Thyroid, Blood Sugar, and Metabolic Syndrome." http://chriskresser.com/thyroid-blood-sugar-metabolic-syndrome.

Last, Walter. "Lipase and the Fat Metabolism." http://www.health-science-spirit.com/lipase.html.

Leibel, R. L., M. Rosenbaum, and J. Hirsch. "Changes in Energy Expenditure Resulting from Altered Body Weight." *New England Journal of Medicine* 332, no. 10 (March 9, 1995): 621–28. doi:10.1056/NEJM199503093321001.

Livesey, G. "Energy Values of Unavailable Carbohydrate and Diets: An Inquiry and Analysis." *American Journal of Clinical Nutrition* 51, no. 4 (April 1, 1990): 617–37.

"More Is Less." *This American Life.* http://www.thisamericanlife.org/radio-archives/episode/391/more-is-less.

Parker-Pope, Tara. "The Fat Trap." *New York Times*, December 28, 2011. http://www.nytimes.com/2012/01/01/magazine/tara-parker-pope-fat-trap. html.

Pick, Marcelle. "Eating To Support Your Adrenal Glands." Women to Women. http://www.womentowomen.com/adrenal-health-2/eating-to-support-your-adrenal-glands-2/.

Sircus, Mark. "Magnesium, Leptin and Obesity." DrSircus.com. http://drsircus.com/medicine/magnesium/magnesium-leptin-obesity.

Swithers, Susan E. "Artificial Sweeteners Produce the Counterintuitive Effect of Inducing Metabolic Derangements." *Trends in Endocrinology and Metabolism* 24, no. 9 (September 2013): 431–41. doi:10.1016/j.tem.2013.05.005.

Taubes, Gary. "What Really Makes Us Fat." *New York Times*, June 30, 2012. http://www.nytimes.com/2012/07/01/opinion/sunday/what-really-makes-us-fat.html.

The George Meteljan Foundation. "Chromium." http://www.whfoods.com/genpage.php?tname=nutrient&dbid=51.

Triantafyllou, A. O., E. Wehtje, P. Adlercreutz, and B. Mattiasson. "How Do Additives Affect Enzyme Activity and Stability in Nonaqueous Media?" *Biotechnology and Bioengineering* 54, no. 1 (April 5, 1997): 67–76. doi:10.1002/(SICI)1097-0290(19970405)54:1<67::AID-BIT8>3.0.CO;2-W.

Triveti, Bijal. "The Calorie Delusion." *NewScientist* 2717 (July 18, 2009): 30-33.

U.S. Food and Drug Administration. "Product Safety Information - Steroid Hormone Implants Used for Growth in Food-Producing Animals." http://www.fda.gov/animalveterinary/safetyhealth/productsafetyinformation/ucm055436.htm.

"U.S. Weight Loss Market Forecast To Hit $66 Billion in 2013." PRWeb. http://www.prweb.com/releases/2012/12/prweb10278281.htm.

Wang, Z., Z. Ying, A. Bosy-Westphal, J. Zhang, B. Schautz, W. Later, S. B. Heymsfield, and M. J. Muller. "Specific Metabolic Rates of Major Organs and Tissues across Adulthood." *The American Journal of Clinical Nutrition* 92 (December 2010): 1369-1377.

Wartman, Kristin. "A Big Fat Debate." Huffington Post. March 4, 2011. http://www.huffingtonpost.com/kristin-wartman/a-big-fat-debate_b_831332.html.

Chapter 7

Brady, Linda J., Daniel D. Gallaher, and Frank F. Busta. "The Role of Probiotic Cultures in the Prevention of Colon Cancer." *The Journal of Nutrition* 130, no. 2 (February 1, 2000): 410–414.

Campbell-McBride, Natasha. "Cholesterol: Friend Or Foe?" Weston A. Price Foundation, May 4, 2008. http://www.westonaprice.org/health-topics/cholesterol-friend-or-foe/?qh=YToyOntpOjA7czoxMToiY2hvbGVzdGVyb2wiO2k6MTtzOjEyOiJjaG9sZXN0ZXJvbHMiO30%3D.

Coscia, Grace Suh. "Can Pickles, Sauerkraut and Fermented Foods Make You Healthier?" Huffington Post. February 1, 2012. http://www.huffingtonpost.com/grace-suh-coscia-lac-diplom/fermented-foods_b_1220756.html.

Dong, Faye M. "The Nutritional Value of Shellfish." 2001 (revised 2009). http://www.wsg.washington.edu/communications/online/shellfishnutrition_09.pdf.

Drum, Ryan. "Medicinal Uses of Seaweeds." 2014. http://www.ryandrum.com/seaweeds.htm.

Fallon Morell, Sally. "Nutrition and Mental Development." Weston A. Price Foundation, June 19, 2010. http://www.westonaprice.org/health-topics/nutrition-and-mental-development/.

Jacobs, Jeremy M., Aaron Cohen, Eliana Ein-Mor, and Jochanan Stessman. "Cholesterol, Statins, and Longevity from Age 70 to 90 Years." *Journal of the American Medical Directors Association* 14, no. 12 (December 2013): 883–88. doi:10.1016/j.jamda.2013.08.012.

Kadooka, Y., M. Sato, K. Imaizumi, A. Ogawa, K. Ikuyama, Y. Akai, M. Okano, M. Kagoshima, and T. Tsuchida. "Regulation of Abdominal Adiposity by Probiotics (Lactobacillus Gasseri SBT2055) in Adults with Obese Tendencies in a Randomized Controlled Trial." *European Journal of Clinical Nutrition* 64, no. 6 (June 2010): 636–43. doi:10.1038/ejcn.2010.19.

Koss-Chioino, Joan, and Philip J. Hefner, eds. *Spiritual Transformation and Healing: Anthropological, Theological, Neuroscientific, and Clinical Perspectives*. Lanham, MD: AltaMira Press, 2006.

Mercola, Joseph. "Health Benefits of Eating Organ Meats." Mercola.com. http://articles.mercola.com/sites/articles/archive/2013/12/30/eating-organ-meats.aspx.

Mielke, M. M., P. P. Zandi, M. Sjögren, D. Gustafson, S. Ostling, B. Steen, and I. Skoog. "High Total Cholesterol Levels in Late Life Associated with a Reduced Risk of Dementia." *Neurology* 64, no. 10 (May 24, 2005): 1689–95. doi:10.1212/01.WNL.0000161870.78572.A5.

Parker-Pope, Tara. "Unlocking the Benefits of Garlic." *Well*, October 15, 2007. http://well.blogs.nytimes.com/2007/10/15/unlocking-the-benefits-of-garlic/.

Ravnsvkov, Uffe. "The Benefits of High Cholesterol." Weston A. Price Foundation. June 24, 2004. http://www.westonaprice.org/modern-diseases/the-benefits-of-high-cholesterol/.

Singing Nettles Herbal Clinic. "Stinging Nettle Urtica dioica." Singing Nettles Herbal Clinic, August 25, 2011. http://singingnettles.blogspot.com/2011/08/stinging-nettle-urtica-dioica.html.

Stanford School of Medicine. "Institute for Stem Cell Biology and Regenerative Medicine: Research." http://stemcell.stanford.edu/research/.

The George Meteljan Foundation. "Omega-3 Fatty Acids." http://www.whfoods.com/genpage.php?tname=nutrient&dbid=84.

Tonegawa, Masanori. "High Levels of Cholesterol Said Better for Longevity." http://phys.org/news203844242.html.

Wade, Nicholas. "Your Body Is Younger Than You Think." *New York Times*, August 2, 2005. http://www.nytimes.com/2005/08/02/science/02cell.html.

Xu, Kevin, MEBO International. July 19, 2013, 2:19 pm. "Humans' Ability To Regenerate Damaged Organs Is At Our Fingertips." *Business Insider*. http://www.businessinsider.com/how-regeneration-works-2013-7.

Chapter 8

Gaesser, Glenn A. *Big Fat Lies: The Truth about Your Weight and Your Health*. Updated ed. Carlsbad, CA: Gürze Books, 2002.

Hurdle-Price, Lynne. "Lynne Hurdle-Price at TEDxWomen 2012," 2012. http://www.youtube.com/watch?v=ZMkQi8aPk6c&feature=youtube_gdata_player.

Jou, Chin. "Counting Calories." Chemical Heritage Foundation. http://www.chemheritage.org/discover/media/magazine/articles/29-1-counting-calories.aspx?page=3.

Keller, Kathleen, ed. *Encyclopedia of Obesity*. Thousand Oaks, CA: Sage, 2008.

Nett, Beth, Joseph A. Brosky, Lynnuel Velarde, David P. Pariser, and David A. Boyce. "Selected Musculoskeletal and Performance Characteristics of Members of a Women's Professional Football Team: Application of a Pre-Participation Examination." *North American Journal of Sports Physical Therapy* 5, no. 1 (February 2010): 1–15.

Reiff, Dan W. *Eating Disorders: Nutrition Therapy in the Recovery Process*. Gaithersburg, MD: Aspen Publishers, 1992.

Taubes, Gary. "Is Sugar Toxic?" *New York Times Magazine*, April 13, 2011. http://www.nytimes.com/2011/04/17/magazine/mag-17Sugar-t.html.

Chapter 9

Ballard, Tom. "Water: The Fourth Food Group." *Sound Consumer*, PCC Natural Markets. August 2005. http://www.pccnaturalmarkets.com/sc/0508/sc0508-water.html.

Chilton, Floyd H. *Inflammation Nation: The First Clinically Proven Eating Plan to End the Secret Epidemic*. London: Simon & Schuster, 2006.

Drum, Ryan. "Sea Vegetables for Food and Medicine." March 2014. http://www.ryandrum.com/seaxpan1.html.

Calbom, Cherie. "The Surprising Truth about Saturated Fats." *Sound Consumer*, PCC Natural Markets. February 2006. http://www.pccnaturalmarkets.com/sc/0602/sc0602-saturatedfats.html.

Environmental Working Group. "Top Tips For Safer Products." http://www. ewg.org/skindeep/top-tips-for-safer-products/.

Fallon, Sally, and Mary G. Enig. "The Skinny on Fats." Weston A. Price Foundation. http://www.westonaprice.org/health-topics/the-skinny-on-fats/#benefits.

Hoyert, Donna L. "75 Years of Mortality in the United States, 1935-2010." *National Center for Health Statistics Data Brief,* 88 (March 2012).

Linus Pauling Institute. "Micronutrient Information Center: Essential Fatty Acids." 2014. http://lpi.oregonstate.edu/infocenter/othernuts/omega3fa/.

-----. "Micronutrient Information Center: Micronutrients and Skin Health." 2011. http://lpi.oregonstate.edu/infocenter/skin.html.

Mercola, Joseph. "The Cholesterol Myth That Could Be Harming Your Health." August 10, 2010. http://articles.mercola.com/sites/articles/archive/2010/08/10/making-sense-of-your-cholesterol-numbers.aspx.

Rose, G. A., W. B. Thomson, and R. T. Williams. "Corn Oil in Treatment of Ischaemic Heart Disease." *British Medical Journal* 1, no. 5449 (June 12, 1965): 1531–33.

Rostan, Elizabeth F., Holly V. DeBuys, Doren L. Madey, and Sheldon R. Pinnell. "Evidence Supporting Zinc as an Important Antioxidant for Skin." *International Journal of Dermatology* 41, no. 9 (September 2002): 606–11.

Sears, Barry. *The Anti-Inflammation Zone: Reversing the Silent Epidemic That's Destroying Our Health.* New York; Enfield: ReganBooks, 2006.

Taubes, Gary. "Is Sugar Toxic?" *New York Times Magazine,* April 13, 2011. http://www.nytimes.com/2011/04/17/magazine/mag-17Sugar-t.html.

University of Toronto. "Some 'Healthy' Vegetable Oils May Actually Increase Risk of Heart Disease." ScienceDaily. www.sciencedaily.com/releases/2013/11/131111122105.htm.

Chapter 10

Blaicher, W., D. Gruber, C. Bieglmayer, A. M. Blaicher, W. Knogler, and J. C. Huber. "The Role of Oxytocin in Relation to Female Sexual Arousal." *Gynecologic and Obstetric Investigation* 47, no. 2 (1999): 125–26. doi:10075.

Carmichael, M. S., V. L. Warburton, J. Dixen, and J. M. Davidson. "Relationships among Cardiovascular, Muscular, and Oxytocin Responses During Human Sexual Activity." *Archives of Sexual Behavior* 23, no. 1 (February 1994): 59–79.

Castleman, Michael. "Four Effective Ways to Break Out of Sexual Ruts." July 15, 2012. http://www.psychologytoday.com/blog/all-about-sex/201207/four-effective-ways-break-out-sexual-ruts.

Ensler, Eve. "Love Your Tree." Interview in *America the Beautiful*, documentary film written and directed by Darryl Roberts. Sensory Overload Productions, 2007. http://www.youtube.com/watch?v=UEUsbLNAfW0&feature=youtube_gdata_player.

Freedman, D. S., T. R. O'Brien, W. D. Flanders, F. DeStefano, and J. J. Barboriak. "Relation of Serum Testosterone Levels to High Density Lipoprotein Cholesterol and Other Characteristics in Men." *Arteriosclerosis and Thrombosis: A Journal of Vascular Biology* 11, no. 2 (April 1991): 307–15.

Frohlich, P.F. and C.F. Meson. "Evidence That Serotonin Affects Female Sexual Functioning via Peripheral Mechanisms." *Physiology and Behavior* 71 (2000): 383-393.

Greenblatt, James M. "Low Cholesterol and Its Psychological Effects." June 10, 2011. http://www.psychologytoday.com/blog/the-breakthrough-depression-solution/201106/low-cholesterol-and-its-psychological-effects.

Grewen, Karen M., Bobbi J. Anderson, Susan S. Girdler, and Kathleen C. Light. "Warm Partner Contact Is Related to Lower Cardiovascular Reactivity." *Behavioral Medicine* 29, no. 3 (2003): 123–30. doi:10.1080/08964280309596065.

Heinrichs, Markus, Thomas Baumgartner, Clemens Kirschbaum, and Ulrike Ehlert. "Social Support and Oxytocin Interact to Suppress Cortisol and Subjective Responses to Psychosocial Stress." *Biological Psychiatry* 54, no. 12 (December 15, 2003): 1389–98.

Horsten, M., S. P. Wamala, A. Vingerhoets, and K. Orth-Gomer. "Depressive Symptoms, Social Support, and Lipid Profile in Healthy Middle-Aged Women." *Psychosomatic Medicine* 59, no. 5 (October 1997): 521–28.

Kaplan, J. R., C. A. Shively, M. B. Fontenot, T. M. Morgan, S. M. Howell, S. B. Manuck, M. F. Muldoon, and J. J. Mann. "Demonstration of an Association among Dietary Cholesterol, Central Serotonergic Activity, and Social Behavior in Monkeys." *Psychosomatic Medicine* 56, no. 6 (December 1994): 479–84.

Kershaw, Sarah. "A Viagra Alternative to Serve by Candlelight." *New York Times*, February 10, 2010. http://www.nytimes.com/2010/02/10/dining/10erotic.html.

Lawson, Elizabeth A., Laura M. Holsen, McKale Santin, Erinne Meenaghan, Kamryn T. Eddy, Anne E. Becker, David B. Herzog, Jill M. Goldstein, and Anne Klibanski. "Oxytocin Secretion Is Associated with Severity of Disordered Eating Psychopathology and Insular Cortex Hypoactivation in Anorexia Nervosa." *Journal of Clinical Endocrinology and Metabolism* 97, no. 10 (October 2012): E1898–1908. doi:10.1210/jc.2012-1702.

Melis, M. R., and A. Argiolas. "Dopamine and Sexual Behavior." *Neuroscience and Biobehavioral Reviews* 19, no. 1 (1995): 19–38.

Mercola, Joseph. "Low-Protein and Low-Carb Diet May Slow Alzheimer's Disease." Mercola.com. March 31, 2013. http://articles.mercola.com/sites/articles/archive/2013/03/31/diet-may-slow-alzheimers.aspx.

Nelson, Tammy. *Getting the Sex You Want: Shed Your Inhibitions and Reach New Heights of Passion Together*. Beverly, MA: Quiver, 2008.

Rerkpattanapipat, P., M. S. Stanek, and M. N. Kotler. "Sex and the Heart: What Is the Role of the Cardiologist?" *European Heart Journal* 22, no. 3 (February 2001): 201–8. doi:10.1053/euhj.1999.2010.

Sabatier, Nancy, Gareth Leng, and John Menzies. "Oxytocin, Feeding, and Satiety." *Frontiers in Endocrinology* 4 (2013): 35. doi:10.3389/fendo.2013.00035.

"Sex Differences In The Brain's Serotonin System." ScienceDaily. http://www.sciencedaily.com/releases/2008/02/080213111043.htm.

"Sexuality and Relationship Online Conference." Conference transcripts. Institute for Conscious Sexuality and Relationship, May 12-16, 2014. http://sexualityandrelationshipconference.com/.

Steegmans, P. H., A. W. Hoes, A. A. Bak, E. van der Does, and D. E. Grobbee. "Higher Prevalence of Depressive Symptoms in Middle-Aged Men with Low Serum Cholesterol Levels." *Psychosomatic Medicine* 62, no. 2 (April 2000): 205–11.

Tuana, Nancy. "Coming to Understand: Orgasm and the Epistemology of Ignorance." *Hypatia* 19, no. 1 (2004): 194–232.

University of Rochester Medical Center. "Omega-3 Fatty Acids and Coronary Heart Disease." http://www.urmc.rochester.edu/encyclopedia/content.aspx?ContentTypeID=1&ContentID=3054.

Wener, Richard and Gary Evans. "The Impact of Mode and Mode Transfer on Commuter Stress, The Montclair Connection." 2004. http://www.utrc2.org/publications/impact-mode-and-mode-transfer-commuter-stress-montclair-connection.

INDEX

ABOUT THE AUTHORS

Jennifer Adler is the founder and owner of Passionate Nutrition, a nutrition practice that uses food—not supplements—as medicine. Passionate Nutrition is the largest and fastest-growing nutrition practice in the nation. Jennifer is a nutritionist, teacher, and speaker, and specializes in helping clients decrease their inflammation, combat depression, prevent and treat cancer, reverse diabetes, manage their weight, and completely reboot their lives through food. Jennifer's philosophy emphasizes abundance and enjoyment over restriction; her approach has been called "the anti-diet." She is a nutritionist with a Master of Science in Clinical Nutrition and Counseling, co-founder of the International Eating Disorders Institute, and has been an adjunct faculty member at Bastyr University since 2006. She holds a graduate certificate in Spirituality, Health, and Medicine from Bastyr University and was trained at the School of Natural Cookery in Boulder, Colorado. Jennifer and the counselors at more than twenty offices take in-person, telephone, and video appointments with clients worldwide.

Jess Thomson is a food writer and recipe developer who has struggled for more than a decade with lupus nephritis, an autoimmune disease that causes fatigue, skin problems, and kidney damage. Following this book's recommendations while writing it, Jess was able to significantly decrease the types and dosages of medications she takes, and also applied some of the methods to help her young son, who has mild cerebral palsy. Jess is the author of six cookbooks, including *A Boat, a Whale & a Walrus*, written with Renee Erickson, and *Pike Place Market Recipes*; her work also appears in magazines nationwide. Find out more about her experiences blending food and life at her blog, *Hogwash*, at JessThomson.com.